fat
church

fat
church

Claiming a Gospel of Fat Liberation

ANASTASIA E. B. KIDD

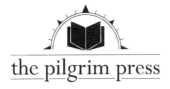

the pilgrim press

The Pilgrim Press, 1300 East 9th Street
Cleveland, Ohio 44114
thepilgrimpress.com

Published 2023.

Printed on acid-free paper.

Library of Congress Cataloging-in-Publication Data on file.
LCCN: 2022939065

ISBN 978-0-8298-0003-6 (paper)
ISBN 978-0-8298-0004-3 (ebook)

Printed in the United States of America.

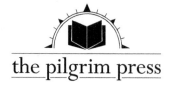

the pilgrim press

Cover art by Bailey Bob Bailey
Book design by Meredith Pangrace

For Cora, in hope.
For Nancy, in gratitude.
For Mona, in love.

CONTENTS

Section Three: Imagining Fat Church

SECTION ONE:

FIRST THINGS FIRST

You probably do not consciously define your life's purpose according to the Myth of Thinness. If asked what you most value, the list would most likely include things like God, your health, love and compassion, inner peace, and your family. Few of us would respond that the size and shape of our figure is what truly matters.

But in our everyday thoughts and actions, the possibility of being thinner may in fact function as our most cherished value and most precious ambition.

—Michelle M. Lelwica [1]

PROLOGUE:

WELCOME TO THE PARTY

Fat Church is the book I have needed to write for two decades, but until recently had neither the gall nor the research to do. I, like most white American women,[1] believed my culture's fatphobic hype and read it directly back onto my own body.

"Fatphobia" is defined by researcher and fat[*] activist Charlotte Cooper as "the fear and hatred of fat people."[2] This may seem a deeply personal descriptor of anti-fatness. No one but the most heinous online trolls, disgusting "men's rights" bros, and draconian personal trainers would ever admit to actually *hating* fat people, right? Right. If queried, I imagine most folks would say the fat *itself* is to be hated, to be feared, to be controlled, not the people beneath it.

But this is basically a "love the sinner, hate the sin" mentality, an all-too-familiar refrain within Christian churches. Just ask any gay person who's attended a "welcoming" but not fully open and affirming congregation. These churches worship under a banner that might as well say, "Sure, you're welcome here. You can worship alongside us. But never forget that there's something fundamentally wrong with you. And that you must repent and change yourself to be fully reconciled with God." Any welcome is filtered through the eyes of judgment and misunderstanding, leaving it at best hollow and at worst overtly abusive.

Over time, queer folks have rejected this paternalism and made spaces for themselves (aided sometimes by their allies) to be known as good, and whole, and an equally beloved creation of God *just as they are*. And thank God for this. Thank God for the fact that just because someone "others" your personhood in the name of religion, that doesn't make it true. And thank God that LGBTQIA+

---

[*] "Fat" is not a bad word, nor is it an epithet. When I use "fat" here I am doing so with neutrality. I will discuss the power of language and reclaiming the word "fat" as a descriptor in Chapter 2.

folks have found or established church spaces where they are not only welcome but affirmed. Having once been ostracized, queer clergy often brightly light the way toward God's love and justice for all people. Having known what it's like on the outside of acceptance, queer people of faith have built social, political, and spiritual infrastructures to better align church and society toward their inherent self-knowledge that God's Creation is full of diverse sexualities, gender expressions, and loving relationships.

It's time for fat people of faith (and their allies) to do the same work of self-discovery, activism, and space-making, so that we, too, can understand ourselves as good, and whole, and an equally beloved creation of God *just as we are.* Yes, just as we are. Each chin and roll a welcome delight in the eyes of God.

So, welcome to the anti-paternalism party, the one where we break the "love the sinner, hate the sin of fatness" piñata all over the dance floor and redistribute the sweetness inside to all bodies who need to finally taste candy without feeling guilty about it.

The guest list starts with people who "struggle with their weight," in whatever form that takes. You're invited to the party if you feel "sinful" or "unhealthy" or "out of control" just because of your body shape. Come and sit, friend, and rest from the idea that you need to lose part of yourself to be good enough. Put down the yo-yo diets that never really work anyway and pick up a cocktail. Give yourself a chance to luxuriate in the idea of never counting another calorie, point, or ketone ever again. And if that makes you anxious, don't worry. You have a long history of radical fat activists, writers, and researchers making a community around you. Keep reading.

Next to be invited are any folks whose bodies are deemed "other" in society, because the struggle for fat liberation is necessarily concerned with your liberation, as well. Fat liberation cannot happen without ending the racialization, ageism, sexism, poverty, patriarchy, and capitalist hierarchy of "productive bodies," all of which keep everyone but the most elite white people impossibly striving. Pull up a chair and know that it's okay if you aren't yet convinced by my argument that fat people deserve a place at the intersection.[3] You have every right to be suspicious of me, given that I am a white, middle-aged, upper-middle-class, cisgender woman. The good news is that there are writers of every hue, social location, and human diversity writing in the field of critical fat studies. Let me introduce you to the broad points and then please seek out their important words.[4] Because individual voices and stories are vital. Fat embodiment—like the experience of any other human diversity—is not universal but particular. Keep reading.

Finally, any person with a body is invited to this party. (I hope I bought enough chips.) Because weight stigma affects all people, regardless of body size. The medicalized weight-loss industry has made sure of this, spending billions of dollars to ensure that we all equate fat people with wastefulness, gluttony, laziness, stupidity, unhappiness, and untimely death, regardless of whether there is conclusive research evidence to support these stereotypes (spoiler alert, there isn't). Weight *stigma* is to blame for many of the negative health outcomes that society turns back onto fat people themselves, gaslighting perfectly healthy fat folks into pathologies that damage both their physical and emotional well-being. *If you care about systemic oppression, you need to start caring about fat people.* Contrary to popular opinion, fat people are not oppressed by their own adipose tissue but by a well-funded, intentional structure of anti-fat bias that has been marketed mercilessly for the past fifty years.[5] One which serves the very weight-loss companies, diet drug pharma, and ob*sity[¥] clinicians who created the fatphobic hype in the first place, and whose profits grow as long as societal hatred of fatness continues to grow. Keep reading.

Whether your body is small or large, aged or young, tall or short, abled or disabled, toned or soft, lithe or stiff, or somewhere in-

---

¥ The word "obese" is a medicalized slur used to make fat people into a disease, which is why it will be typed with an asterisk. See Chapter 2 for a further discussion of ob*sity as a word and concept.

between these dichotomies, anti-fatness affects us all because it is *intended* to. None of us is impervious to the near-constant barrage of anti-fat imagery surrounding us. It arises in all forms of media and is so casual that it has become imperceptible to most. Who among us laments the weight stigma inherent when a fat character is slovenly, sexless, lazy, or eats an overly large sandwich for laughs? These stereotypes are just accepted as funny. Millions of us watch "thinspiration" like *The Biggest Loser* and *My 600-lb Life*—shows expressly developed to exploit fat people for monetary gain, just like the carnival sideshows of yore. We moralize our food using language like "good," "bad," and "cheat day." We buy into diet programs, which knowingly use the caloric equivalent of starvation and are tantamount to eating disorders, and then blame ourselves when our bodies do not have the "willpower" to adhere to that abuse for more than a few months. We allow our children to be weighed at school using an equation made up by a nineteenth-century Belgian mathematician (not physician) that has been repeatedly debunked as a scientifically meaningless measure of fatness (yep, the BMI is pure horse pucky[6]) and that stigmatizes young people into body shame, to lasting effect.[7] We make New Year's resolutions to "be better" and "try harder," to make "lifestyle changes" that will finally stick. They never do. We punish, restrict, and use all sorts of measures of control against our bodies' expansion to make sure they don't transgress certain size boundaries. We deny ourselves fleshy pleasures in ascetic performance of how important it is to maintain as close proximity to culturally defined perpetual "perfection" as possible.

We all do these things. I do them, too. I just do them less than I used to because I've learned so much about how anti-fat hate was manufactured, and how it functions to perpetuate even more anti-fat hate. It's a pretty efficient little economy, too. I got off that hamster wheel, at least as much as I can. I'm still working on it, to be honest. It's really hard to pull away from something so insidious as commercialized diet and beauty culture and the medicalized weight-loss industry. But I'm one-hundred-percent done being a self-hating, ever-dieting puppet of fatphobic marketing, actively lining the pockets of my oppressors with my hard-earned money. I'm onto new things, like learning to listen to my body and trusting its cues to tell me what to eat and when. Like eschewing the fear of death that has hung over my fat body like a phantom funeral pall my entire youth, in favor of living life as best I can for as long as I can. Like allowing myself pleasures of food, sex, and other embodied practices without shame, as if I deserve good things in this fat body. Because I damn well do. We all do.

So, pull up a chair and join the Fat Church party. Listen carefully until you hear the echoes of fatphobic injustice that may not initially seem to affect you directly but, my God, most certainly do.[8] For we are all involved in what religious scholar Michelle Lelwica calls "The Religion of Thinness,"[9] a moral code written on US society that functions with its own set of beliefs, rituals, and myths to keep fat bodies (and so many others) oppressed.

And here is where I want to specifically invite Christians to the party, particularly those of the more "liberal-leftist-progressive" ilk. Fat Church takes for granted that #BlackLivesMatter, queer people are beloved, and that Jesus was not only reorienting his people toward God but standing up against an empire. If you haven't yet closed this book after that sentence, pull up a chair. They're sturdy and armless. Because it's time for the Christian church to take up the cause of fat liberation as one of the intersectional spaces necessary for social justice.

This book is for fat people, particularly female-identifying and femme people of all genders and expressions, who are told in myriad ways that they must live up to unattainable standards of beauty, health, and wellness without being told that these same standards are rooted in racism, capitalism, and patriarchy.

This book is for trans folks whose gender confirmation surgeries are put on hold until they reach a certain BMI, their doctors forcing them into unsustainable diet practices before they can rightfully live in their most authentic bodies. I am so sorry this is happening to you. Don't blame your good body for this fatphobic medical cruelty.

This book is for parents whose own internalized anti-fat bias will inevitably affect their children's idea of self-worth and justice for others.

This book is for the person who won't be photographed, erasing their very visual history in order to avoid commemorating their girth.

This book is for every person who hopes they are currently a "before" picture to some imagined "after" where they will finally be satisfied with the weight or shape of their body.

This book is for young people, so that they may learn lessons about their belovedness decades before I did and begin healing from the inherited generational trauma that is manifested as hatred and fear toward fat bodies.

This book is for naturally thin people who believe the maintenance of their body shape is equivalent to the maintenance of the body shapes of their more corpulent neighbors, and thereby judge fat folks' inability to "control" themselves.

This book is for "out-of-control" fat people, so they might examine what it means to put their bodies "in control" in the first place, and whether this is a worthy goal at all.

This book is for fat people in the midst of, or recovering from, eating disorders that their doctors and friends will never actually believe they have because they "look" well-fed.

This book is for people whose bodies have not yet become fat but will in middle age. For the paunches and love handles and muffin tops to come. May they be welcomed as a natural and beloved part of aging, fascinating shifts brought about by complex metabolism and genetics, rather than feared.

This book is for formerly fat people who have achieved their "best bodies" by diets and exercise. Perhaps you are one of the two percent of people who can keep the weight off the rest of your life,[10] and perhaps you are not. Either way, your body is amazing for all it has already done. It will be no less amazing if it gains weight again someday.

This book is for those who have had costly bariatric surgeries and are in lifelong stages of recovery. May you treat your body kindly as you reorganize your relationship to food and society and not become an evangelist for something others may not have the stomach to do.

This book is for me because its lessons have been hard-won over a lifetime of struggle to reach past self-hate, past even self-love, to a place of fat advocacy that seeks freedom for all bodies that are marginalized.

This book is for you, because no matter who you are, I guarantee you know something about fat and hold some internal judgments about it. Welcome to the party.

This is not a self-help book, though I hope that some might find it helpful. It's also not a simple "God loves you just the way you are" text. I do believe that is true, but saying or even trusting the truth of that statement does not fix the numerous spiritual, emotional, and physical problems arising from US culture, which has a fanatical fascination with fitness, places moral worth on body size, and demands penance to purge the sin of fatness. There is something soul-wrenchingly dangerous about the way Americans deal with the intersections of body, weight, gender and race, sexuality, economics, and spirituality. *Fat Church* hopes to contribute to the fat activist conversation from a progressive Christian standpoint. Hopefully, it will help shed light on the often unseen anti-fat bias we encounter and perpetuate every day as Christians, so that we might start new conversations about what it means to be fat and faithful in the church and wider society.

Finally, it's the fact of my own fatness that gives me a sense of urgency to do this work, born from the ways my body interacts with the world each and every day. While all people can struggle with their bodies in a capitalist system that demands they do so, living in a body labeled "morbidly ob*se" since childhood has given me particular and painful insight. For this reason, this book includes a bit of memoir, because to talk about body oppression in a disembodied way is not only inauthentic—it also serves to reinforce the notion that such issues can be decoupled from the bodies on which they feed and inflict pain.

Stories of how individuals experience anti-fat bias in our lives, even in the church, are meant to express the urgency with which body liberation should be collectively sought. People are in real pain and will continue to be unless change happens. All of us need to hear fat peoples' stories to be able to consider how they interact with our own. Hopefully, they will incite solidarity in instances where another's story sounds intimately familiar. At other times, these stories will be completely "other" and yet no less true and worthy of reflection. Perhaps some who read this book will begin to realize their own culpability in perpetuating body oppression, whether upon their own or others' bodies, and will join the movement toward body liberation and fat appreciation as a means of repentance.

All the personal stories in this book, though told individually, are meant to highlight a collective truth: that the way we feel about our own bodies, and talk about them privately and publicly, has collective power. It is important to realize that *when we as individuals participate in our own fatphobic behavior or rhetoric, it doesn't just hurt ourselves*. When we hear how anti-fat bias affects all people, perhaps it will resonate in a way that fuels action. We may seek justice for others that we would never be brave enough to seek for ourselves. We may hold our tongue from its usual people-watching judgments. We may begin to see the strength and resilience and beauty in fat people, rather than stereotypes of shame.

Presenting stories is also a means of combating the image of the "headless fatty," the decapitated fat body, filmed from the neck down, that treads across our screens whenever America's "ob*sity epidemic" becomes the focus within the media.[11] You know these images from the evening news or accompanying popular magazine articles about the latest diet craze. They're often shown eating or drinking, reinforcing the stereotype that fat people can't stop gorging ourselves. These bodies are filmed this particular way and placed as specimens for public ridicule because of their fatness, with their faces blurred or cut off entirely in an effort to keep their anonymity. This is, at best, a misguided attempt to prevent the fat person's embarrassment (as if someone wouldn't notice their own clothing onscreen), or more likely a self-serving ploy to avoid legal action for publishing someone's photo without permission. But in every case, those fat, headless bodies are not just dehumanized symbols but whole people—their faces and minds as well as the stories they share and memories they hold.

So, when I share from my own story, or quote from someone else's, it's for the sake of reminding us that there is no such thing as disembodied weight bias or opinions about one fat body (even one's own) that do not directly affect every other fat body. Stories from marginalized bodies of any kind become vital to the work of their anti-oppression. And one's own body liberation must necessarily root itself in the systemic dismantling of body oppression for all. At least if it's to do any lasting good.

The purpose of *Fat Church* is to help us all examine our anti-fat judgments, hold them up to the light of medical, historical, and theological inquiry, listen to and believe the narratives of fat people, and hopefully emerge understanding the vital need for radical fat acceptance within and beyond the church as a part of God's intersectional movement toward body liberation for us all.

Now where is that piñata?

CHAPTER 1:

A BIG FAT CHILD OF GOD

What is the good news for fat bodies?

This is a necessary question. We tend only to hear bad news about fatness. We hear statistics and slurs and jokes and advertisements that all seek to make sure that those of us who are fat believe wholeheartedly that we are failures. This is why fat folks are very much in need of good news. And it's why *all* people need to be saved from their anti-fat hatred and fear of adipose tissue by a gospel of fat liberation.

As I write, I am an ordained United Church of Christ minister who weighs around 350 pounds, and who has thoroughly traversed the "ups and downs" of living in a fat body within the social location of white, American[1] Christianity. And yet, in many ways, this book is my first public admission to being a fat person.

This will seem like a strange statement to anyone who has ever met me. There is no doubt, peering at the cut of my jib, that my body is hugely, impressively fat. I almost always take up more physical space than anyone else in the room. My corpulence has been my most constant companion and my most prominent defining feature; my body the biggest frenemy I could imagine throughout my life. I have lived in simultaneous shame and awe at my size. I have oscillated between times of self-hatred and self-acceptance, usually winding up in the mire of rebellion against a phantom perception of who I "should" be physically.

For years, I thought this rebellion was against "fatness" itself and all that it supposedly meant. My body was fat, sure. But what I was mostly trying to avoid were the attributes so often culturally conjoined with "fat." Things like fat-and-*lazy*, fat-and-*unhealthy*, fat-and-*ignorant,* fat-and-*ugly,* fat-and-*smelly,* fat-and-*selfish.* Thus, I tried to keep the blatantly obvious fact of my weight a peripheral trait, something that didn't define me. I would be hard-working, healthy, educated, pretty, perfumed, and selfless. I would be enough of all the things that "fat people" are not to make both me and others forget that I was fat. But nothing was enough.

I hate to admit it now that I know better, but being fat made me feel like an absolute and total failure. No matter what I accomplished, I did it while fat. And I believed this was an obvious sign that something was amiss with my personhood and/ or moral willpower. It was exactly how author and researcher Brené Brown speaks about shame as a constant cycle, an emotion difficult to understand but pervasive (especially in women) and used to great effect in our culture. As she says: "You work hard to show the world what it wants to see. Shame happens when the mask is pulled off and the unlikable parts of you are seen. It feels unbearable to be seen."[2] I wore my biggest shame like several down jackets in the summertime—heavy, obvious. To my mind, it eclipsed everything else I did, so I worked hard to shine brighter than my body, to be The Nicest Person, The Funniest Person, The Most Compliant and Selfless Person. And when I failed because no one can be nice, funny, compliant, and selfless all the time, my shame was compounded.

My shame was not a failing of my self-confidence or even faulty logic, considering the lifetime of anti-fat messages I digested from the media, American medicine, and even my own beloved family and friends. Fat people are invited, almost required, to believe terrible things about themselves in a culture that labels them an epidemic. A contagion. Fatness is unreservedly ridiculed, shamed, and demonized, and so it makes sense that I bought into this fatphobic fearmongering and aimed it inward. I was right where the seventy-eight-billion-dollar weight-loss market[3] wanted me—fat and unhappy about it, clinging to the life raft diet fads they sold, trying to escape the very cesspool of fat shame they had spent millions of marketing dollars creating in the first place.

Then my Mama died.

Mama was the absolute best, most loving parent one could imagine—an idyllic Donna Reed-type homemaker who was the very definition of womanhood for me as a child. And I learned from her that part of what it meant to be a woman was wrapped in the performance of "beauty." Mama was conventionally beautiful throughout her life. She was blonde-haired, blue-eyed, and curvy but svelte until later middle age, which is when I came to live with her. Mama and Papa were my paternal grandparents, and they spent their "golden years" raising me after my birth parents' contentious divorce. During her fifties and sixties, Mama gained weight despite her best attempts not to do so.

Mama was perpetually dieting, and, as her chubby daughter, we went on these diets together. I stirred the pot while she chopped the vegetables for our "miracle cabbage soup" diet. I inventoried our pantry, discarding anything with too many carbs, as she made an Atkins-friendly grocery list. Mama cut our every-morning grapefruit in half and I sprinkled the juicy, pink segments with Sweet'N Low. Together we measured out portions on our kitchen scale and calculated the "exchange points" for our dinner plates. Dieting was our constant hobby, and yet, by the late 1990s, Mama had peaked in her weight as a size 18. I remember her frustration as a personal dig since I was already a size 20. Dieting made Mama and I co-conspirators against our supposedly unruly bodies, and I thought the never-ending struggle to be smaller was part and parcel of what it meant to be a beautiful, though never-beautiful-enough, woman.

Mama fought metastatic breast cancer for about a decade before succumbing to it in 2013. Always impeccably coiffed, she lost all her treasured blonde hair to chemotherapy. A brain tumor made one of her sky-blue eyes involuntarily close. And her body grew thinner and thinner as her sickness progressed. She was unnaturally small, her body frail, and her appetite nil. I tried to convince her to eat whatever she wanted, whatever she could stomach amidst her nausea. One day she commented on how she found it strange that she was craving peanut butter. "Oh my gosh, then eat some! Have a couple spoonfuls each day! That'd be great protein for you!" I implored. "No, no. There's too much fat in it," she replied.

No matter how much she withered, Mama continued to pour skim milk onto her low-carb, high-fiber cereal, even though it went untouched save for a bite or two. The more robust nutrition of whole milk would be an unthinkable splurge. A 100-calorie pudding cup became too filling for one sitting. "I wish I had this kind of willpower before now," she quipped, and we laughed together sadly. At the end, Mama wore the size 6 of her young adulthood, finally back to her goal weight on her deathbed. She died at home wearing a size "small" pair of pajamas. She was surrounded by loved ones. I was holding her hand.

Something in the loss of my mother, and in her final weight loss, broke my fat shame. Something in the way she refused foods that might have brought her some physical caloric strength, or even just joy, in her last days, infuriated me. I simultaneously grieved the tremendous loss of the woman I most idolized and the realization that weight loss had become her idol, and therefore my idol, as well. Encountering her death up close, I reflected on how much of her life was spent unsatisfied with her body, determining daily success on the basis of numbers on a bathroom scale or the fit of an old pair of pants. I loved my mother with every part of my being. With her gone, it was time for me to love my fat body like she never could hers.

It has taken me almost a decade to move from grieving daughter, still dutifully counting my calories, to fat activist, counting on fat liberation.

I began to research "fat" both as a biological truth and a cultural concept. I wanted to understand what fat is, to become acquainted with this huge part of me. For too long I had bought into the dieting cliché that said I was a thin person trapped inside a fat body. I thought of my fatness as a temporary state, something I intended to eliminate and thus never cared to get to know. But what if my fat was never problematic surplus? What if it's just me?

I intentionally began to imagine myself as "fat," not as a temporary but a permanent state. This mental shift itself was absolutely revelatory. "This is my identity. I am a fat person." I said this over and over in my mind, trying to make it stick after a lifetime of promising myself eventual thinness. I started trying out the word "fat" as a neutral self-identification. I stopped thinking of myself as a "before" to some imagined "after."

At first this mental shift toward claiming fat identity felt like giving up, an acquiescence rooted in my failure to control my big body and bend it toward thinness. But soon I realized that this perpetual self-critique was a lie born of the diet culture that promises, with just a bit more willpower or a new monthly membership, I can be freed from my fat forever.

Here I must say that my hope of thinness was only ever a straight-up Ursula K. Le Guin-meets-Neil Gaiman fantasy. I now laugh at diets promising to help me regain my thigh gap or lose my love handles. I'm not going to tame my copious belly with a thirty-day Slim Fast liquid diet or "cayenne cleanse" juicing regimen. To become a medically "normal" weight, my body would need life-threatening levels of intervention.[4] I'm always going to look more like Venus of Willendorf[5] than Venus Williams. I have been fat literally my entire life and most of my biological family members have been fat when they weren't dieting.[6] So, why did I perpetually imagine that I could become such a different body type? What sustained this unattainable fantasy? One guess—it rhymes with "weight-loss industry." All seventy-eight billion dollars of it. Aimed right at my sense of self-worth.

I bet I am not alone. We have all seen the magazine covers with newly thin folks stepping easily into one leg of their enormous pre-diet jeans. We've heard the "success stories," seen the "after" photos of dangerous-but-clearly-worth-it bariatric weight-loss surgeries, right? *The Biggest Loser* is a popular US television phenomenon and "thinspiration" to millions of viewers. And so, I held on to my fantasy of thinness until I could not do so anymore. Until the enormous shame of never actually attaining the fantasy became heavier to bear than both the real and imagined weight of my own fat body.

But the truth is: I am fat, and that is not going to change.

Embracing that fact has been a blessing. Through my own learning, I started to recognize that the vast majority of what makes my fatness difficult is societal. It's difficult receiving inadequate and dismissive health care from my doctors. It's difficult being jeered on the street from passing cars or "secretly" photographed on public transit. It's difficult having fewer, more expensive stores in which to shop for clothes. It's difficult being fat on an airplane or in theaters, with seatmates audibly angry at my proximity. It's difficult having to constantly fight against the stereotypes of my fatness to earn people's kindness and respect, especially knowing that, even when I manage to earn it, their judgments likely remain. My body doesn't fit into society's norms or, quite literally, its chairs. But my bruised thighs and bruised ego are actually one and the same, suffering not from being fat but from a culture deeply disinterested in my thriving as a fat person.

I came to realize over time that my former defiance at being defined as "fat" was not so much a denial of my obvious body type, but rather pointed against the untruths that are written by society onto fat bodies. Fat people can be (in fact, most are!) productive, self-controlled, and happy. Fat people are beloved, desired, and have great sex. Fat people can be content with their bodies just as they are and not want to be one ounce thinner. And fat people have existed, and thrived, all throughout history.

These facts were once revelations to me as I emerged from the depths of my own internalized anti-fat oppression into the open air of fat activism. The internal whisper that my fat body is whole and good, even great, grew louder as I voraciously read blogs, journal articles, and whole histories of fat cultural emergence. I hoarded these books like a dragon discovering treasure for the first time, filling one, two, three bookshelves. There were fat autobiographies and collections of essays in critical fat studies readers, books on the social development of the healthcare industry over centuries and its simultaneous public health trends, biology texts on the complexity of fat as an important endocrine organ of the body, histories on the cultural emergence of beauty along with subsequent feminist and womanist critiques, moral philosophy and virtue ethics, liberation theologies, queer and crip theory,[7] gender and sexuality studies, poetry and prose in praise of corpulence, and inspiring recounting of six audacious decades of organized fat activism ("We're here! We're spheres! Get used to it!"[8]). With so much of the media's focus being on eradicating fatness, I was amazed that simultaneous research existed on *positive* fat identity. And it all pointed toward the right for fat people to exist unmoored from societal shame.

Fat activism is important for the lives of fat people, yes, but also for many more.[9] There is generational trauma in how we perpetuate and enact anti-fat bias onto the bodies of our children. And the struggles of fat people to gain acceptance are inextricably bound up with the thriving of other socially oppressed and minoritized groups. The struggle for fat people to not be objectified or assigned value based on their proximity to culturally mandated "beauty standards" aligns with the struggle of all women under the gaze of patriarchy. The struggle for fat bodies not to be medicalized and understood as unnatural aberrations aligns with the struggles of trans and queer people to be seen as inherently of sacred worth. The struggle for fat people to enjoy unequivocal dignity and civil rights rather than death-dealing policing aligns with the goals of the #BlackLivesMatter movement and others in racialized communities. The struggle against fat eradication as a people aligns with the struggle of Indigenous communities under continued industrial and political colonization. The struggle to make society an easier place for fat bodies, with all the spatial accommodations necessary to move freely and exist in public without pity or ridicule, aligns with the goals of many in the disability community. And the struggle of fat people to carve out of their societal oppression a sincere love for themselves and a life-affirming society in which to thrive is the struggle of all marginalized folks.

The power of the Christian gospel has always been its invitation to organize society in a new way. The church can choose to use this power for either colonization or liberation. Through a gospel of fat liberation, we can reorder society toward communal wellness that does not rely on a hierarchy of bodies. We can end structural health disparities. We can remove anti-fat judgments of ourselves and others. We can enjoy the bodily delights of food, movement, sex, and even swimming without intrusive thoughts of personal shame. In this way, salvation comes, not with yet another diet regimen, but with our deep-down belief that there is beauty, dignity, and value inherent in all bodies, of every size, even in our own. Jiggles and all.

All of this begins with claiming our fat identity—permanent, unapologetically positive fat identity. This is how a gospel of fat liberation grows: by naming fat people a powerful community rather than weak individuals. By seeing God's incarnation at work in our bodies just as readily as anyone else's. By living the truth of our belovedness as big, fat children of God.

God's welcoming embrace is large enough for bodies like mine. It does not demand that I shrink into worthiness. My size is not a sin nor is my fatness indicative of a lack of faithfulness. This truth is one facet of a more broadly gleaming gospel that says the good news of God's welcome extends to all bodies everywhere. After all, Jesus's earthly ministry regularly favored those with marginalized bodies that didn't fit into society's norms.

If spread, this good news can liberate fat people from the damning internal judgments of constant comparison. It can liberate us from the perpetual cycle of restrictive diets that never last. It can liberate us from the inferior healthcare and personal-responsibility narratives that threaten our lives. And it can build loving communities around those of us who are isolated from society due to our size.

This is a gospel that must be understood to be spread, and the misinformation about fatness is legion. So, take a breath and get cozy. Here we go. And may we, the Fat Church, shape our beliefs, politics, and actions toward a world in which the gospel of fat liberation spreads as easily as warm butter.

CHAPTER 2:

THE "F" WORD

I am fat. This statement is a neutral marker of my identity. I would tell you with the same amount of neutrality that I am above average in height for an American woman,[1] my hair is greying in fabulous shocks at my temples, I wear a size 11 shoe, and I prefer glasses over contact lenses to correct my nearsightedness. Why is it that, among these truths about my body, fatness strikes such a negative chord?

People engage in all manner of verbal Olympics to avoid the term "fat" because of the emotional power of that word in our society. Bullies use it to take down their prey. Marketing agents use it to arouse fear or disgust in order to sell us their products. Real housewives whisper it behind one another's backs. And when we say it about ourselves, "fat" rarely has a positive connotation.

This is why here, at the very beginning of this book, we need to discuss the power of reclaiming the word "fat" as a neutral marker of personal identity, no more a moral failure than being "tall" or "brunette." Because to be afraid to say that one is fat—and choosing instead fluffy, big-boned, plump, chubby, husky, poofy, zaftig, Reubenesque, corpulent, thick, or fleshy—is a reminder that to be simply "fat" is something bad and worthy of disdain.[2] One can be as "curvy" as they'd like to be, but there is liberation in owning the term "fat" just as easily.

I say nonchalantly that I am fat. It rolls off my tongue naturally without inherent judgment. But this was not always so. It took me a good, long while to stop using all the other synonyms for "fat" as cute little smokescreens of contempt for the fat on my own body or on the bodies of others. It took years, in fact, of unlearning the negative messages I inherited from society about fat in order to say this tiny, three-letter word painlessly. If you are reading this bewildered that anyone could claim fatness as a positive identity marker, I invite you to similar unlearning. I wrote this book for you.

Yet all of the condescending niceties for avoiding the word "fat" are far preferable to the medicalized language we place on big bodies. "Ob*sity" as a word is intensely offensive, so much so that you'll notice I've chosen to write it with an asterisk as a visual cue that this word is a slur to fat people like me. Trust me when I say that this is a pain-in-the-butt way of having to type this word out each time, and fat activists wouldn't do it if it wasn't a completely necessary action. For my part, I will only use the full word "obese" herein when it's quoted in another person's writing because I don't feel I can change their words as they intended them. But even just now, typing that extra "e" gave me a shudder.

"Fat" is a neutral word for adipose body tissue that will be used liberally throughout this work, while "ob*sity" is a word that originates in anti-fat bias. The word comes from the Latin phrase *obedere*, which means "to overeat," or "to eat oneself to the point of fatness." Thus, there is inherent individual blame attached to the word ob*se. It automatically assumes the origin of fatness is personal gluttony, which (as we will see) is rarely anyone's simple truth.

The word "ob*se" was used in literature as a mocking term for fat people for centuries before it suddenly became a medical description of fatness in the mid-twentieth century. Researcher Thomas Baldwin described this problem in a presentation to the World Health Organization saying:

> Taking a derogatory term and seeking to repackage it as
> a descriptive medical term is undesirable. For it is bound
> to be heard as a way of stigmatizing those to whom the
> term is applied. It's as if the terms "stupid" and "stupidity"

were taken from their current derogatory use and used to describe the condition of those with some mental handicap that leaves them with a very low IQ.[3]

Imagine modern medicine repackaging the study of those with developmental disorders as "Stupidity Studies" and you will have a sense of how "Ob*sity Studies" sounds to someone like me, someone who is trying to neutralize and even celebrate fat identity. Those who would like to become more adept allies to fat liberation are invited to reclaim the word "fat" and avoid "the o-word" as much as possible.

Fat liberation is another term that demands early defining. Fat liberation is not the liberation of bodies *from* their fat. Oh no, not at all. It's the liberation of all bodies—fat, thin, and everything in-between—from rampant diet culture and the not-good-enough-ness it forces onto perfectly good people, as well as the "fat panic"[4] it breeds in society. It also seeks to liberate the narrative of fatness away from medicalized notions of disease back into the hands of fat people themselves, understanding them as agents worthy of both dignity and voice.[5]

In this way, fat liberation is a political movement[6] that seeks rest from the century-long battle in American society to erase and eradicate our fat bodies. This work puts fat activists in solidarity with other embodied political movements seeking safety, civil rights, and dignity. After all, much of this country's fondness for thinness is inextricably intertwined with its history of white supremacy, body policing, colonialism, and capitalistic determination of whose bodies are most "valuable" in society (see chapter 5).[7] What we think about "ob*sity" in America isn't just about fat. It's about power, and politics, and money, and social scapegoating, all under the guise of "health." That, to me, is what gives anti-fat hate its particular *chef's kiss* *je ne sais quoi* of complete bullshit.

Though it may seem impossible, there is another way to engage fatness. You may have noticed the power of this alternative at work through increasingly positive visual representations of fat bodies in popular media; the spread of #bodypositivity and "Health at Every Size" movements; the rise in social media stars like Dexter Mayfield (@dexrated) and Anna O'Brien (@glitterandlazers); and the popularity of podcasts such as Aubrey Gordon's and Michael Hobbes' *Maintenance Phase,* which already is listed among Apple podcasts' "Top 100" shows less than a year after its launch.[8] Affirmative engagements with fatness spread because they strike an emotional chord for so many who have been told that their fat is a problem to be solved and a weakness originating in poor willpower. These alternative narratives are full of eye-opening truths about how the diet industry works against *all* bodies, especially the most marginalized,[9] and how "personal responsibility" ideals of wellness undermine the public health of all but the most monied elite.

These emerging fat acceptance trends find their origins in the decades-long history of the fat liberation movement. Much of the early history of fat activism is lost to time, but some intrepid fat activists, like Charlotte Cooper,[10] have produced DIY archives of personal papers, audio-visual recordings, photos, and timelines.[11] This has prompted the growth of "fat studies" as its own critical field of inquiry over the past twenty years, with exponential growth in published research since the 2010s.[12] Here the use of the word "critical" connotes a commitment to criticize and interrogate existing societal structures and their underlying assumptions rather than taking society's anti-fat bias for granted (like ob*sity studies do). Fat studies are "critical" in the way they look under the hood of fatphobia to see how its engine was built—with the hope of dismantling it for good.

Critical fat research and fat ethnography directly counter much of the work of medical ob*sity studies. While ob*sity studies pathologize fatness as a disease and seek the eradication of fat people by weight loss,[13] fat studies understand fatness as a valid body type and use body size as an identity lens through which to criticize any number of societal oppressions. For those interested in the latest research, *Fat Studies* is an interdisciplinary, peer-reviewed journal published three times annually by Taylor & Francis since 2012. It provides a repository of much of the fat studies scholarship happening today.[14] However, true to its roots in 1960s queer culture, fat activism continues to develop on the margins, outside the pages of academically acceptable readership, in blogs, zines, websites, and chat rooms. This is where the action is, the work of real people navigating the ambiguities of living in an already-but-not-yet time of fat acceptance.

But who gets to claim the word "fat" as part of their personal identity? This is an important question when even svelte celebrities and Olympic gymnasts are fat shamed.[15] The request to "picture a fat person" inevitably conjures a spectrum of sizes in our minds. There is a helpful taxonomy of fatness originating with Ash Nischuk, the host of *The Fat Lip Podcast*, known as the "Fatness Spectrum."[16] While most medical charts categorize fat bodies using the BMI or other problematic measures of ob*sity,[17] Nischuk's spectrum relies mostly on the more neutral descriptor of clothing sizes. Using United States' sizing standards, she identifies "small fat" as those wearing a US size 18 or lower (corresponding to sizes XL or 2XL), "mid fat" as sizes 20 to 24 (corresponding to 2XL or 3XL), "superfat" as sizes 26 to 32 (corresponding to 4XL to 5XL), and "infinifat" as sizes 34 and higher, who often cannot shop for clothing in stores and must find custom-sized fashion options online.[18] Instead of saying "normal weight" to indicate someone thinner, the term "straight sized" is better, as it does not imply a normative weight for which people should strive.

These characterizations are helpful in fat discourse since fatness is nuanced and experiences of oppression are not the same across the fatness spectrum. For example, most "body positivity" and "weight inclusive" health initiatives have focused on small- to mid-fat bodies, leaving superfats and infinifats still on the margins. And while access to compassionate and thorough healthcare, adequate clothing, and size-inclusive representation in the beauty and health industries have started to improve for those at the lower end of the fatness spectrum over the past decade, there is still much room for improvement in services and support at the larger end of the spectrum. This is why superfat and infinifat bodies are often centered in the politics of fat activism. Without their inclusion there can be no true fat liberation.[19]

Here I want to say just a quick word to my peers: white, affluent, progressive American Christians who earnestly want to live into the idea that God's welcome and love is for all of Creation. We try our best, we do. And yet we are so entrenched in the systems of injustice, racism, privilege, and capitalism that to free ourselves from these bonds is a lifetime effort from which we will not likely emerge victorious. Yet and still, it is a vital duty to remain engaged in the struggle for freedom from all oppressive systems, whether or not we benefit directly from that struggle. Do not get tired or complacent. Others don't get to enjoy the privilege of disengaging, so neither should we. Anti-fat bias is rooted in all of the other systems of injustice and must be addressed as well. The struggle for God's love and justice to be known on earth must include an understanding of all bodies, at all sizes, to be seen as sacred and worthy of that love and justice now. Not "one day" or "when they've lost the weight," but now. Right now.

While on the surface this may seem an easy mantra to take up, like all forms of justice, its realization in day-to-day living is much more difficult. It is extremely complex, this un-weaving of the way one feels about her own body, the way society has been built to make her feel about her own body, and the way the Christian church has been complicit in (and in many ways actively contributed to) her body oppression.

How many of our Christian "ideals" around "health and wellness" (read: thinness) mirror society's own desire for lithe and youthful figures? Where does "your body is a temple" theology end and the capitalistic self-hate weight yo-yo begin? How do the historical Protestant pieties of "moderation," "temperance," and "purity" intersect with body policing of all sorts? Why have women's bodies been particularly monitored for adherence to beauty, health, and wellness standards throughout the Christian story? We will ask these questions and more together.

CHAPTER 3:

DANGEROUS BUT LIBERATIVE UNLEARNING

What is written herein is an invitation to unapologetic, liberative fatness—a fatness unconstrained by what society would deem "appropriate." This is a fatness that wears white, especially after Labor Day. This is a fatness that speaks up in pride when others try to shame it. This is a fatness that fights back with a fierce inner light of worthiness as its holy guide.

And I'm in a dangerous position as I write this manuscript.

This is because I consider myself a fat activist. I try to live unapologetically as a fat person in society and I fight for the rights of others my size and larger to do the same. I'm concerned not only with fat assimilation (that is, the acceptance of fat people into mainstream culture as equally valued citizens) but true body liberation, with its wider political goals of freedom from body policing of any sort, as well as full and equitable dignity for people of all sizes, shapes, ethnicities, and human diversities.

And yet, I'm also writing this book as a primer, an introduction for those who have never been disavowed of the lies of diet culture and its pervasive hold on the medical and media industries in our country. I'm writing most particularly to progressive American Christians who don't realize that some of our faith tradition's theological underpinnings have functioned to create and sustain anti-fat hatred and the denigration of bodies outside of upper-class white Protestantism. I'll need to offer a certain amount of foundational research for this audience to begin to notice, question, and maybe even start to dismantle the anti-fat bias in their midst.

So, I'm in this quandary that will make both the fat activist and the diet culture novice uncomfortable.

Radical fat activists will see me fall into assimilationist traps of using research to challenge what is meant by "health" and offering statistics to suggest fat people are not, on the whole, different from their thinner counterparts save for their negative experiences with diet culture and rampant medicalization. Though all of this is true, it's politically unhelpful for fat people seeking body liberation to focus solely on these truths. Because these truths are pitched toward the too-basic goal of fitting fat folks into American society as dignified humans rather than avatars of presumed disease. I do want that. My God, do I want that. But I also know that any arguments that center what Kathleen LeBesco calls "fat innocence"[1] (things like "We can't help it! We don't eat any more than you do! We can be healthy at this size!") undermine both fat political power and personal agency, replacing them with bland supplication for fat people to be seen as "normal." This is an unhelpful practice of fat respectability politics.

Historian Evelyn Higginbotham coined the term "the politics of respectability" in 1993 as a way of describing how some Black women chose to self-present in a way that challenged prevailing racist stereotypes for the sake of gaining access to the white-controlled middle-class society.[2] Those who downplayed their Black identity in order to "fit in" found more welcome in white society than did others. However, in exchange, these women's full humanity was always being negotiated within the realms of white supremacy. "Respectability" could reap individual benefits for those willing to play that game, but it did nothing to change the systemic structures that denigrate Blackness as a whole.

Since then, critics of respectability politics have noted their twofold danger. Respectability politics reinforce in-group stratification between those who act "respectable" and those who reject such presentation. The "pull up your pants" discourse in Black community politics is an often cited example of this.[3] And respectability performances also reinforce the notion that ethnic embodiments either unfamiliar or problematic to white culture can and should be eschewed. "Just because white people do not like our behaviors doesn't mean they're not perfectly good behaviors," critics of racialized respectability politics rightfully say.

In a similar way, fat people do not need to shoehorn themselves into medicalized diet culture by proving their proximity to "health," nor make their bodies perform respectability by eating only dressingless salads in public, wearing conservative clothing, or even avoiding society altogether. The goal of fitting into "normal" American society is a pretty low bar when what you *really* want to see is the dismantling of white supremacist neoliberal capitalism and its usury effect on bodies of all sorts. Whew! That's a big idea with words that may not yet make any sense, but they will by the end of this book.

Those who are entirely new to thinking about the ravages of diet culture on society might imagine some of the arguments of this book to be extreme:

- The everyday things we do and say about our own and others' fat have wider societal implications.
- The medicalized wellness industry doesn't have fat people's best health interests in mind but rather their own pocketbooks.
- The medicalization of fatness as a disease arose in nineteenth- and early twentieth-century pseudoscience rooted in white supremacy and is sustained primarily by neoliberal capitalism.
- Seeing fat people as a disease could lead to their eugenic medical genocide.

- Unapologetically embracing one's fatness can be a revolutionary way of embodying anti-capitalism.
- Fat is a good, even desirable form of embodiment.
- Traditional theologies of the Christian church are at work in this country's cultural anti-fatness.
- We can begin to heal our relationship to fat bodies with a spirituality that emphasizes the goodness of all Creation instead of the doctrine of Original Sin.
- And the most extreme argument of all: God created fat bodies to be just as they are.

This is what you're here for, so get ready.

Odds are that this book will make you angry at times and incredulous at others. It may create a sense of guilt or embarrassment at being duped by pervasive yet false anti-fat narratives. It will press on unseen bruises and the reactions may be sharp pains of denial. Because fatness is something we supposedly know all about. We know that fatness is unhealthy and leads to an early death. We know that gluttony is a sin and that all fat people are gluttons at heart. We know that fatness can be changed with a simple equation of calories in/calories out. We know that anyone who wants to be thinner can lose weight if only they have the willpower to do so. Here's the thing: every one of those claims is false.[4] We will interrogate them all.

The challenge of such ingrained anti-fat "knowledge" means that we must unlearn much of what we've been taught to be true about health, wellness, and their equation to moral goodness. This unlearning *should* be an emotionally fraught exercise. For me it has felt something akin to the feeling I have when growing in my knowledge of white supremacy's hold on this country. When I learned, for example, that the "ob*sity epidemic" was created as an intentional marketing ploy by the diet industry and has been promoted by the medical industry for financial gain,[5] this had an emotional impact on me. And my subsequent anger grew in me a combination of righteous indignation and commitment to change similar to my commitment to antiracism.

Here I must take care not to equate the evils of slavery and colonization with anti-fat hatred. They are not equivalent. While societal oppression of fat people is extreme and widespread, we fat folks have not been systematically rounded up and forced into physical labor like those who were enslaved and removed from their homelands. I am not making that comparison here and pray I will never have the opportunity to do so.

Yet anti-fat rhetoric is continually rising in this country,[6] often as a proxy for racism itself.[7] Some public health authorities already suggest shaming and punishing fat people for their size alone.[8] Public health laws targeting ob*sity are increasing.[9] Doctors are allowed to refuse to care for patients above a certain BMI and health insurance companies routinely deny coverage above a certain weight limit.[10] Weight-based discrimination is legal in 49 out of 50 states.[11] And social media is full of debates like "If it was a law for fat people to lose weight immediately, would that be a bad thing?"[12]

The hope of fat activists (and their closely aligned disability rights counterparts) is that the vitriol and scapegoating of fat people might retract. However, these acts of discrimination seem to be growing to a potentially ominous, yet still unknown end. This fact puts pressure on including anti-fatness as yet another systemic oppression that we must dismantle to have any hope of a truly liberative society. And the Christian church must be taken to task for its philosophies that underlie anti-fatness the same way we critique those beliefs that propped up slavery and genocide.

Yes, this is dangerous work and much is at stake within it. But far more dangerous is believing in the personal responsibility narratives of health that are quick to damn anyone who becomes unwell. We must rely instead on what Sonya Renee Taylor reminds us is true: "the body is not an apology."[13] Fat people have nothing for which they must apologize, and it's time we stop living like we do.

THE COOKOUT

I sat at my family cookout, happy to be in the company of my parents, husband, aunt and uncle, and chubby eight-year-old cousin, who was noshing on his second hamburger of the meal. "You must be hungry tonight!" someone said to him, followed by, "growing boys need their protein!" "He's such a good eater," admired another, "maybe he'll grow up to be a football player." My young cousin smiled and reached for the ketchup.

I couldn't help but contrast this scene with my own experience, many years before, of being eight years old and chubby, and being weighed in front of my mother's Weight Watchers friends, all of whom treated me like the cutest little mascot of their group. I didn't have a goal weight, not really. There was a number that my "coach," or company representative, had chosen for me from a matrix of age, height, and weight. Since the chart began at age sixteen, she had to guess for me, and it was finally decided that my goal weight should be what my coach's own, "normal-sized" granddaughter weighed, since we were the same eight years old.[1] I needed to lose forty-two pounds.

While others were weighed in private, I would approach the scale with a gaggle of eager women around me, hoping the best for me—that I would have lost a pound or two over the past week. If I had, I would be treated to all the accolades: "You're really doing great! Way to go! You'll be to your goal weight in no time!" If I gained weight that week I was treated to the group's wisdom: "You need to try to exercise; you get recess, don't you? Why don't you run laps during recess?" Many times, I received the most foreboding advice of all: "You better lose it now, or you're never going to. You don't want to go through life fat. You'll die young." That comment single-handedly introduced me to the existential threat of death. Thanks, Sharon.

From the weigh-in, we as a group moved to the classroom where, my feet not touching the floor from my chair, I would be advised to substitute low-fat cottage cheese with a little sugar-free applesauce on top if I was craving ice cream. Even with the imagination of a child I couldn't make that one work out.

Back at the cookout, my mind was wondering about my own complicated relationship with food when I was my cousin's young age. To be honest, at that moment I became a little jealous of him, with his cute and chubby face all full of second-burger delight. It was at that very moment that I—at the time a twenty-eight-year-old woman who had lived her entire life in a fat body—understood that there was an intersection of gender and body size, and that, as a woman, I was on the wrong societal side of it.

I was instantly transported back to my own eight-year-old self. Back then, instead of "growing boys need their protein," it was, "little girls shouldn't eat so much." And "he's such a good eater!" became, "should she be eating that?"

I shook myself out of my memories, reaching for another burger in defiance. I ate every bite of it, even though I was already full.

My cousin has since grown to be a downright skinny man in his early twenties, while I have continued to put on weight, fueled by the habits of body shame and restrictive dieting that I learned early in life. Weight Watchers in my aughts gave way to Nutri-System and the dangerous diet drug Fen-Phen in my teens, pursued alongside weight-loss therapies such as biofeedback, hypnosis, and even an overnight trip to Memphis's Le Bonheur Children's Hospital to make sure my thyroid wasn't acting out in some way that could explain why I was fatter than all my peers.

I remember receiving the answer that I had no thyroid issues as a disappointment.

SECTION TWO:

ANTI-FAT BIAS, ITS ORIGINS, AND ITS CONSEQUENCES

Fat activism isn't about making people feel better about themselves. It's about not being denied your civil rights and not dying because a doctor misdiagnoses you.

—Cat Pausé [1]

CHAPTER 4:

THE PREVALENCE OF
ANTI-FAT BIAS

The headline hits me during an aimless midnight scroll through Twitter. A South African woman living in New Zealand since 2018 has applied with her family for citizenship and has been denied on the basis of her weight.[1] At 282 pounds, she is deemed by the government to be a financial risk to their country's socialized medicine. She will not gain access, even despite the fact that doctors and medical tests agree she has no actual health problems. Still, she is determined to lose the weight for the sake of her family of four, who are all stymied in immigration limbo until she does. I make a prediction. She will not be able to do this on her own but will be forced into bariatric surgery, forever changing her relationship to food and her body. She will gain access to New Zealand, now thinner but permanently medicalized. Their prediction will come true. Her body will become their medical burden.

I weigh a lot more than this woman does. And so, at 12:14am on a warm June night I suddenly become too fat for New Zealand. The world just got a little smaller for my big body. I know not to read the comments on this article because I'd like to sleep tonight. I keep scrolling.

A court just removed two fat teenagers from their family home because of their failure to lose weight, which the court deems grave child abuse. The local government had provided a free gym membership, Fitbit movement trackers, and Weight Watchers meetings, so clearly any failure was willful on the family's part. After the court hearing that placed the teens in long-term foster care, the judge lamented her own decision, but said it had to be made so the kids might "learn ways of living more healthily."[2] She offered: "The case was such an unusual one because the children had clearly had some very good parenting, as they were polite, bright, and engaging."[3] Thank goodness she got these clearly well-adjusted teens into the loving embrace of the foster care system to learn that their politeness, brightness, and engaging personalities matter far less in this world than their physical size. I pause to pray for them that they might know their belovedness. I pray for their devastated parents. I pray for an end to weight-loss culture and its dehumanizing effects.

Maybe I should just stop reading Twitter. Maybe "The Algorithm" is showing me heinous anti-fat stories because for the past five years I've spent much of my time researching systemic anti-fat bias and the negative effects of weight stigma. When you search for "fat activism" as much as I have, these articles might just be the aftermath. I Google fatness so much that the word "fact" often autocorrects on my phone. That's a fat.

Anti-fatness exists all around us in American culture where diet, beauty, and medical industries consort with one another, and the fat body—especially the fat female and femme body—is considered a failure of them all. I am tired of this narrative and the way it harms people. I am no longer shocked at the prevalence of anti-fat hate and how often it shows up as a supporting character in modern American life, especially alongside misogyny and white supremacy. I'm just shocked that we Christians aren't talking about those connections more or trying to do something about them. Especially as people of faith. Especially when the headlines keep coming.

Weight-based stigma was used as a primary defense in the 2021 trial of Derek Chauvin, the police officer who murdered George Floyd.[4] Though it did not prevent Chauvin's being found guilty, the "ob*sity defense" prevailed in the trial of the 2014 killing of Eric Garner in New York. Defense attorneys argued in both cases that Floyd's and Garner's fatness contributed to their deaths by choking,[5] so police brutality should be let off the hook. In the case of Eric Garner's homicide, the "ob*sity defense" worked. The officer responsible for his death was not convicted despite using a chokehold banned by the NYPD[6] and despite his ignoring Garner's eleven cries of "I can't breathe." Turning to the media to validate the verdict, US Representative Peter King (R-New York) reflected the defense's argument back to the CNN audience, saying: "If he had not had asthma and a heart condition and was so obese, almost definitely he would not have died from this."[7] Anti-fatness ultimately shapes public discourse about anything that happens to a fat person, even their own death.

Anti-Fat Bias in Right-Wing America

Social media is often where anti-fatness thrives unchecked. In the fall of 2020, a social media analysis of white supremacist hate-group culture uncovered clear links between their alt-right brand of hyper-masculinity, racist Western "pride," and weight stigma, which fat activists had long observed anecdotally.[8] Private messages obtained surreptitiously from the Patriot Front—a fast-growing militant hate group—showed that "the men, who believe the United States is a nation that belongs only to white people, wear uniforms made up of bomber jackets, face coverings, and beige khakis, mandate weight-loss and intense workouts, and regularly practice hand-to-hand combat."[9] Weight loss is a primary concern because fatness is synonymous with softness and femininity, both antithetical to their ideal that strong white men are needed to defend the "American way of life."

Similar analysis of right-wing popular news coverage shows a conflation of anti-fatness and anti-feminism. Fat hate often stands in for misogyny, and vice-versa, both in articles and in the commentary posted by viewers beneath them.[10] The conservative media maven Ann Coulter captured this fat-feminist hatred in her heinous and widely shared tweet after the 2016 election of Donald Trump. She captions a photo in which a larger woman with a bullhorn fronts a group advocating for the rights of immigrants: "Without fat girls, there would be no protests."[11] Cat Pausé and Sandra Grey offered a fat activist rebuttal:

> What the Coulter tweet demonstrates is that fat women are perceived as doubly-problematic in public space, both as fat and as women. They do not do politics in a way that is befitting womanhood—they are too visible and loud; they are not moral guardians of conservative values; and, their bodies challenge masculine power.[12]

There is a terrifying power in the bodies of fat women, it seems. A power that, to some, must be contained as fat itself must be.

And they're trying. Take for example the $2000-per-ticket, self-proclaimed proudly-misogynistic event called the "Make Women Great Again Conference," also known as the "22 Conference."[13] It gained notoriety for its all-male lineup of speakers and incendiary keynote topics focusing on how women can lose weight and attract a "real" man, have "unlimited babies" while keeping their bodies taut, and know their place "in the kitchen and the bedroom."[14] When, exactly, *were* women great? Well, before feminism ruined us, of course! This is the conference's central message from its website:

> Hiding under a mask of fake progress, feminism today has become a radical assault on all forms of positive femininity—you know, the one hard coded into your DNA. Through an onslaught of anti-feminine propaganda

spanning generations, <u>women today have been pushed to act like men</u> and DENY their own feminine nature. This has left millions of women feeling unhappy, confused, frustrated, and hopeless. At the 22 Convention, you will learn the truth that unhealthy militant feminists have been hiding from you your entire life . . . <u>Men admire healthy, fit women</u>. They are after all sizing you up for reproduction, and your decisions will be passed on to your children through the choices you make via epigenetics . . . High quality masculine men want high quality feminine women to mother their children and set great examples for their daughters. Our speakers will teach you what men and women of prior generations FAILED to teach you as a direct result of feminist meddling and sabotage.[15]

There's so much to unpack and critique. But the message is clear: feminism ruined women, making them fat and unfertile. Through reprogramming, the conference promises women will "raise their femininity by 500%," and its founder believes this will save our country. He warns:

I'll put this in very blunt terms: America has zero future with masculine women and feminine men. None. The consequence of not making women great again will be the total collapse of the American family this century and the resulting collapse of the USA.[16]

The link between women's bodies and their political power is clear again here. And fatness is a symbol of power that these men don't want women to gain.

Those who call ourselves progressives/liberals/leftists understand the racism and xenophobia at work in our white supremacist society, and we see the obvious misogyny promoted by hyper-masculinity and anti-feminism. But we rarely notice the third circle in the "Make America Great Again" Venn diagram—anti-fatness—because this is often the one value we share with them.

Anti-Fat Bias in Left-Wing America

It's still deeply, dangerously counter-cultural to point out fatness at the intersections of oppression, even among the most liberal, welcoming-of-otherness people.[17] But anti-fat bias is culturally in-grained *on both the right and left sides* of the aisle.

Some of the most "woke," culturally competent critical thinkers I know are often unaware of, sometimes even proud of, their own anti-fat bias. They off-handedly equate fatness with Republicans and conservative capitalists, greedy with monied excess. When called out, they don't see the shame at work in their denigration: "Well, they *are* fat! Just look at them." As if the fact of their opponents' undeniable fatness somehow demands comment and ridicule.

Aubrey Gordon describes the pain of seeing #MarALardass and other fat-hating political cartoons aimed at Donald Trump's ample waistline during his presidency.[18] Like me, Gordon is no fan of Trump's politics. But this is not because of his fatness; it's because of his terrible ideologies. And yet his political opponents frequently took cheap shots at his looks, further denigrating all fat people in the process. As Gordon says, "the political Left [has] used the deep-seated fear of fatness to attack opponents, galvanize a base, and symbolize capitalism, greed, poverty, and ignorance."[19] The trope of the fat, dumb conservative with a Southern accent is played over,[20] and over,[21] and over again[22] in liberal spaces, but mostly belies how biased even the "open-minded" really are.[23]

We see this bias in the left's uninterrogated food politics. Many decry fried, fast, and processed foods, lamenting the "food deserts" of some urban, usually non-white communities,[24] but then they direct the full force of their activism toward pop-up farmer's markets. This only does what white supremacy usually does: it reduces systemic social change to matters of personal responsibility. The thinking seems to be: give the poor, brown people the choice of more vegetables and they'll finally be thin and healthy, like elite whites are. Of course, we'd never say this out loud. We may not even realize we're thinking this way. But the motivations *behind* our motivations still matter greatly, because "personal responsibility" is the nexus of racism and diet culture in cahoots.[25]

Fatima Cody Stanford is a Harvard researcher[26] studying the link between what she calls "the two most common forms of bias in the United States . . . race bias, which is by far the most common, followed by weight bias."[27] Stanford notes:

> About 80% of Americans believe people with obesity are primarily responsible for their obesity . . . similarly, a full 50% of white Americans believe that racial disparities in jobs, income and housing can be eliminated if Black people tried hard enough. These personal responsibility narratives aim to convey that the locus of change is at the personal, not the systemic, level.[28]

Systemic change would interrogate and seek to modify the government subsidies behind certain foods, study the effects of pesticides on the body and environment and regulate them, provide weight-neutral healthcare for all, address the root issues of poverty, stop redlining and gentrification efforts that create two unequal economies, and limit the powers of food lobbyists and diet industry leaders who often make our food choices for us. Better than just a farmer's market, no?

And we progressives want all of these things. But we too often couch our "change" in narratives of personal responsibility, seeing fat people as their own problem. Take this horrendously anti-fat, racist, classist conclusion from the horrendously anti-fat, racist, classist article by Greg Crister that was a cover story for *Harper's* magazine entitled, "Let Them Eat Fat: The Heavy Truths About American Obesity"[29]:

> What do the fat, darker, exploited poor, with their unbridled primal appetites, have to offer us but a chance for we diet-and-shape-conscious folk to live vicariously? Call it boundary envy. Or, rather, boundary-free envy . . . Meanwhile, in the City of Fat Angels, we lounge through a slow-motion epidemic. Mami buys another apple fritter. Papi slams his second sugar and cream. Another young Carl supersizes and double supersizes, then supersizes again. Waistlines surge. Any minute now, the belt will run out of holes.[30]

The "primal appetites" and the "un-boundaried spread" language loudly echoes the nineteenth-century newspapers that decried immigrant arrivals and their presumed contagion (see chapter 5). Crister's piece was written in 2000, and much has changed since then, but a lot hasn't. Perhaps an article like this would not be published now. But this kind of thinking is still alive and well all around us. It inspires study after study on "ob*sity in communities of color," and cultural heritage foods are decried as "obesogenic" by researchers who can't even pronounce them correctly. This is all the same American conflation of racial marginalization and anti-fatness, couched in the patronizing "bootstrap" mentality of personal health. Beware the government officials trying to "uplift the urban poor" with free Weight Watchers memberships instead of a minimum wage above the poverty line.

Okay, but what about the progressive folks who understand the problems with making fun of fat people, who celebrate body positivity and human diversity, and who offer a full-throated "yaaass"[31] to Lizzo's[32] ample thighs? Surely, they "get it," right? Sometimes. And other times they have a size limit to their robust inclusion. Some believe they are making room for fat people when they say, "Fat bodies are great (as long as they're healthy)!"[33] As Amy Erdman Farrell offers, "it is as if an invisible line separates the thin-enough feminist who is allowed to critique the excesses of the diet industry from the fat 'other' who resides outside the boundaries of normative citizenship."[34] Progressives may be able to make room for small-fat, medium-fat, and maybe even some superfat people who are otherwise "healthy" (or seem to be at a healthist[35] gaze). But are our politics wide enough for the infinifat, the home-bound fat, and those who most need our systematic efforts toward their accommodation and ample, dignified living? Or is pity and an invitation to the gym the best we can offer?

While progressive circles readily wrestle with other societal "-isms," sizeism is still a relatively new venture for many, particularly white folks who have been both beholden to and benefitted from the societal pressures of diet culture the most. This makes sense. Liberal whites are the ones keeping Whole Foods,[36] Soulcycle,[37] and overall "wellness culture" afloat. And while participation in these brands or the natural food movement may not be *itself* anti-fat, the messages within their origins and marketing[38] certainly are.

"Wellness" as a concept originated in 1970s hippie counterculture and its primary tenets were a distrust of modern Western medicine to provide optimal health, an embrace of non-Western alternative regimens (such as yoga and vegetarian or raw food diets), and a focus on one's personal responsibility for their own health "self-optimization."[39] Journalist Sirin Kale describes how anti-fatness arose within wellness circles:

The polluting tributary in wellness's fresh, clear stream has always been its unwavering insistence that health is a choice rather than something genetically predetermined or socially ordained. Few wellness practitioners say outright that people who are morbidly obese, have type 2 diabetes or have a mental illness suffer by their own hand: they instead couch their judgment in euphemisms and misdirection . . . For nearly 50 years, the world of wellness has viewed health as something that can be shrugged on or off at will, like a cashmere sweater. Doctors are to be distrusted and individuals should take responsibility for their own "wellness journey."[40]

Anti-fatness is an underlying value of wellness brands.[41] And the promise of thinness is part of their mass appeal. This is the hard truth, my progressive friends: any money we pay into wellness brands becomes part of upholding the systemic oppression of fat and non-normative bodies, no matter how well-intentioned we are.

The Political Refrigerator

A mere ten days before the 2020 presidential election, the *New York Times* published an article entitled, "Quiz: Can You Tell a 'Trump' Fridge From a 'Biden' Fridge?"[42] Only about fifty percent of the refrigerators were guessed correctly by the *Times'* readership, but the gallery of the most accurately answered fridges is telling. These play directly into America's weight-based and food-based stereotypes: Republicans as the fat, processed-food eating masses, and Democrats as crunchy-granola lefties hellbent on forcing bland clean eating down everyone's throats. Oat milk vs. Mountain Dew becomes a political choice, not just a personal preference. But, of course, moralizing what we eat is nothing new. We see it every time Guy Fieri pats his adorable paunch at the latest diner, drive-in, or dive, proclaiming "it's cheat day!" before tucking into cheese fries.[43]

Each and every day, in small ways and large, I navigate this strange world in a superfat body, pinball-like, bumping up against anti-fatness in politics, in the media, in medicine, in my church, in everyday conversation with strangers and friends alike. I didn't used to see it. But now that I do, it's obvious everywhere. And it's driven me to believe that ending weight stigma is not just about making the world a better place for fat people, though it would do that. It's a fundamental part of dismantling all the systemic oppressions that undergird our American society.

CHAPTER 5:

WOMEN, WASPS, AND WEIGHT

Historically, family health was considered women's work, part of managing the home.

In their domestic roles, women were tasked with remediating illnesses with folk medicine—home remedies of herbs, tinctures, and ample prayer.[1] Through their cookery and management of family hygiene, women could either introduce and spread sickness, or ward it off altogether. After all, given the medical infrastructure existent in colonial America, one spoiled supper could lead to the demise of an entire household.

With "wellness" a primarily female issue to address, and "illness" a problem for which wives and mothers were often blamed, women became a good market for the burgeoning economy of magazines. Cheaper to print than books, easy to collect and share with friends, women's periodicals proliferated in the colonial era among the elite and middle-class women who could afford them. Those who wrote copy for these magazines quickly took the opportunity to conflate women's care of their own bodies with the care of their household, often dramatically tasking women with the wellness of growing America's "civilization."[2] Thus, articles on body shape and beauty (often synonymous); fashion, health and wellness; food and recipes; and Christian spirituality spread to housewives across the land, shaping a uniquely American cultural ideal of healthy (white, Protestant, upper- and middle-class) womanhood.[3] These magazines made it clear that a woman unable to manage wellness in her own body could not likely manage a household or land or keep a husband. Yes, the conflation of beauty, marketing, and homemaking that still rules women's magazines today is not a new invention in the slightest.

Sabrina Strings describes how the development of "health and beauty" standards in American women's magazines were racially motivated, as well. White European (more specifically, Anglo-Saxon[4]) Protestant "settlers" colonized Indigenous lands in the name of the Christian God. They understood the Native peoples they encountered to be dark-skinned "savages" that they could eradicate, push aside, enslave, and/or deculturate into irrelevance.[5] Through participation in the transatlantic slave trade, the colonists sought the arrival of additional non-white bodies to be forced into labor and grow American prosperity.

Strings illustrates how enslaved Africans were often described in the media of the time as "small" and "greedy," supposed signs of primitivity and gluttony, in clear contrast to the tall, thin, and "controlled" American ideal of Northern European Anglo-Saxon beauty.[6] The nascent American medical industry took notice of these "different" bodies, as well, leaning into the pseudoscience of phrenology and declaring "race" a biological concept.[7] There were public autopsies of enslaved people's bodies, travelogues of the "savageries" experienced while traveling to other lands, and medical sideshows played for public entertainment and financial gain. These spectacles of "otherness" served to dehumanize anyone outside of the white Anglo-Saxon lineage (American society's "norm") and have had lasting effects.[8]

The medical industry still today uses the Body Mass Index (BMI) as a universal standard of "normalcy," despite its origins in nineteenth-century medicine's race-based pseudoscience. A Belgian mathematician and astronomer named Adolphe Quetelet came up with an equation of the ideal weight-to-height in 1832, which was based on his research of white, European men.[9] He described this "average man" in his writings, saying, "if the average man were completely determined, we might consider him as the type of perfection . . . and everything differing from his proportion or condition, would constitute deformity or disease . . . or monstrosity."[10] Even still, Quetelet never intended his equation to be used in medicine, nor for it to be used to measure individuals at all, but rather to measure the shift in collective human proportionality over time.[11] Using it as a marker of individual "ideal" weights was the idea of Ancel Keys, a nutritionist who rose to national fame by working with the US military on the question of starvation. He was hired to determine just how many calories of food were needed to supply those at war. His last name thus became the source for the term "K-rations," the pre-determined amount of food that soldiers fighting in the Second World War were fed each day. This led to the popular perception of Keys as one of this country's great authorities on nutrition, wellness, and health throughout the twentieth century.[12]

Keys began experimenting with fat people in the 1950s. Describing fatness as "ugly," "disgusting," and "repugnant," Keys was trying to find a link between "overweight" and other diseases, but he needed a standard measurement of weight on which to base his studies. He, of course, turned to the natural place . . . nineteenth-century Belgium! And the Quetelet Index, which Keys renamed the BMI, became the universal medical standard of "normal" body weight used in almost every study of weight in this country from that time onward.[13] Many (if not most) in today's medical industry recognize the problematics here, but claim the BMI is too well-established in the research to ever be extracted from use. This is despite the fact that it cannot be trusted as an individual marker of wellness, provides suspect results, and is foundationally racist.[14] (It's even more fun to note how doctors change the BMI measures of "overweight" and "ob*se" from time to time to put more Americans in these categories. This not only increasingly inflates notions of the "ob*sity epidemic" to great public fear and outrage, but conveniently allows these same doctors to bill insurance for more "ob*sity interventions."[15])

Back to colonial America. The most widely distributed home-use medical handbook ever published, William Buchan's *Domestic Medicine,* originated in Edinburgh in 1769 and came to the United States two years later; at least thirty editions were released in this country over the next hundred years.[16] Marketed to women for the proper care of their households, Buchan's *Domestic Medicine* helped define notions of health, wellness, prevention, and cure in early colonial American culture. Buchan did not altogether eschew the notion of doctors for special illnesses, but deemed them unnecessary for treating most diseases, emphasizing instead a daily regimen and "virtues of simplicity" like cleanliness, fresh air exercise, and a disciplined diet.[17] With these and a few home-concocted medicines, Buchan noted, there would be no need to seek the more complicated prescriptions of doctors.

Buchan was not the first to encourage personal responsibility and simple living to assure one's good health. He found his precursor in none other than John Wesley, the founder of Methodism, who in 1747 wrote *Primitive Physic,* a medical advice book that boiled down to much of the same fare as Buchan's.[18] Wesley's ideas about health spread across the country just as his evangelistic "circuit rider" missions did. Part of Wesley's theological method for living a holy life was physical wellness, which he understood to be God's intention for all bodies.[19] Disease, to Wesley, was a function of human sinfulness, and insomuch as someone could ward off illness through "inward and outward health," they would be able to better pursue a righteous Christian life.[20]

Presbyterian minister Sylvester Graham would take up this same charge of pious personal responsibility for health (especially as evidenced by what one eats) as part of his lectures, which began on the anti-alcohol temperance circuit of the 1830s.[21] Growing his popularity and reach as both a religious and pseudo-medical scholar, Graham emphasized that eating flavorful foods and meats led to illness of both body and soul. Only through a strictly weighed diet of bland and easily digestible vegetables, fruits, and grains; cold water; and milk could one achieve physio-spiritual wholeness, he moralized, and followers called "Grahamites" were born all over the country. Sometimes whole institutions, like Oberlin College, followed his flavorless regimen for years at a time.[22]

Graham's lasting culinary legacy can still be found on grocery store shelves everywhere—the Graham cracker. He postulated and preached that those little unleavened golden squares held enough nutrition to stave off a body's unnatural lusts, such as gluttony and masturbation.[23] Yes, to early American Protestant figures like Graham, good health was understood to be one's own responsibility. Insomuch as "sinful" behavior could be avoided, so would health be assumed to follow by the grace of God.

Waves of immigrants arrived on America's shores during the 1800s. The sheer masses of Irish, German, Chinese, Italian, and Jewish people from Eastern and Central Europe threatened the Anglo-Saxon "bloodline"[24] and the Protestant religious establishment in American culture. The immigrants' "strange" foods, curious religious practices, and different bodies were suspect and frequently written about in popular newspapers, magazines, and medical journals.[25] The language of "disease" arose as established White Anglo-Saxon Protestant (WASP) Americans surveyed their new neighbors. Immigrants' diseases soon became a worrying "threat to public health" (though the perceived threat was always much larger than in reality).[26] Still, caricatures of immigrants, often drawn as fat and with visual cues of disease, persisted in popular media. Judith Walzer Leavitt's compassionate biography of Mary Mallon, the Irish immigrant also known by the dubious moniker "Typhoid Mary," provides an example of how real humans were behind all this hysteria. She writes that "the epithet and the woman merge and they are indistinguishable."[27] Xenophobia was quickly dehumanizing immigrants into symbols of disease. And equating fatness with both.

Concerns about public health were a front. What was really at stake was maintaining WASP culture as people mixed with one another, intermarried, and got frisky in the growing cities of late-nineteenth and early twentieth-century industrial America. WASP women's fertility and chastity became of utmost importance to stave off "race degeneracy," which was discussed openly in the medical journals and popular literature of the time.[28] Xenophobic concerns about public health, overt white supremacy, and anti-fat bias thus became inextricably intertwined within elite American society. And dieting became a way for white women to show their commitment to the Anglo-Saxon physical "ideal" (thin but strong) in the midst of a diversifying society.

Yet initially, at the turn of the twentieth century, the concern was that WASP American women were *underweight*, not overweight. Physicians worried that too-thin women would be unable to birth strong Anglo-Saxon children at the same rates as the "immigrant hordes" they feared. Thus, society as they knew it eventually would be upended, with WASPs displaced as America's elite.

This concerned physician John Harvey Kellogg,[29] who concocted[30] a highly regimented vegetarian diet of various grains alongside lots of water, both as a drink and to soak in as baths, to strengthen women for increased vigor and fertility.[31] Dr. Kellogg's plan was so popular that his brother, W.K. Kellogg, would go on to create a food manufacturing empire based on the corn flake cereal that was central to the Kellogg diet.[32]

The goal of John Harvey Kellogg's diet was to create in women an economy of careful balance and bodily control. He called for the suppression of all gluttonous, "animalistic" appetites. This fit both Kellogg's Protestant penchant for moderation and his racist beliefs that non-white people were prone to succumb to their uncontrolled urges.[33] Self-control while eating became a measure of one's "civility," a code word for proper white upbringing. With careful monitoring of nutrition and behavior, all people (but most importantly women[34]) could become their most perfect, God-intended selves.

Kellogg became a major voice in the "clean living movement" that emerged, which was aimed not only at individual health but at staving off "race degeneracy" within society.[35] In 1914, Kellogg co-founded the Race Betterment Foundation in Battle Creek, Michigan, where he also housed his popular health resort, the Battle Creek Sanitarium. Thousands of Americans flocked there to learn how to improve their health and social status through "clean" eating, self-control, and eugenics ("proper" breeding).[36] Kellogg's nutritional writings filled the women's magazines of the time, endorsed by their WASP editors who were similarly inclined. Articles were indistinguishable from advertisements and both sold Kellogg's brand of diet aids. In this way, American diet culture was founded not only to improve one's physique but also explicitly for the continued propagation of white Anglo-Saxon Protestants for the nation's ruling class.[37]

While Kellogg's primary concern was underweight women's fertility failing the Anglo-Saxon "race," others pointed to fat women's bodies as the true race traitor. After all, being fat was a betrayal of the lean Anglo-Saxon ideal form and this made fat women's genetic origins suspect. A chestnut from Edith Bigelow's article "The Sorrows of the Fat," published in *Harper's Bazaar,* offers a glimpse of how outright the anti-fat-meets-racism rhetoric could be within women's magazines circulating at the turn of the twentieth century: "[A fat woman] will not be a social success unless she burnt-cork [blackface] herself, don beads, and then go to that burning clime where women, like pigs, are valued at so much a pound."[38]

Though diet culture began in WASP circles, other women seeking to climb the social ladder eagerly took part and more "fad diets" were born. "Fletcherism" promoted the chewing of each bite of food until it was liquified before swallowing, a slow process that supposedly helped with nutrition and digestion. Weight-loss potions laced with chemicals like arsenic and cocaine sped up the metabolism but also had life-threatening side effects. Women's magazines advertised "sanitized tape worm pills," which were ordered in the hopes a parasite might grow inside one's intestines and absorb their errant fat.

Despite all these interventions, Americans started getting fatter. Industrialization caused increased riches for the middle class, and this, along with the rise of factory farming, allowed Americans to eat fuller meals.[39] At the same time, women started working outside their homes in the mills and factories, changing the way families ate and kitchens looked.[40] Women left their larger, rural houses behind and moved to apartments where kitchens were smaller. Meals had to be more efficient, or store-bought, because women's work schedules afforded them less time to cook. Fashion and beauty also played a role in women's self-understanding of body size "normality." While tailors had once created individual garments for each customer, mass-produced fashions began to be sold in stores, introducing sizing standards that now categorized women: small, medium, and large.[41]

In 1918, Dr. Lulu Hunt Peters produced America's first best-selling diet book, *Diet and Health: With Key to the Calories*. Written and marketed directly to women, Peters introduced a "1,200 calorie schedule" (a nearly fifty percent reduction from the food intake of the average woman at the time) replete with examples of how much of each food equaled hundred-calorie portions.[42] Peters offered suggestions to her hungry female followers of how to remain steadfast on their diets, saying:

> You may be hungry at first, but you will soon become accustomed to the change. I find that dry lemon or orange peel, or those little aromatic breath sweeteners, just a tiny bit, seem to stop the hunger pangs; or you may have a cup of fat-free bullion or half an apple, or other low-calorie food.[43]

For those well-versed in diet culture, this language may sound familiar. Indeed, most diets of the early twentieth century have simply been repackaged and sold to subsequent generations.

Peters' diet book made a special point to equate being thin with patriotism, given that American involvement in the First World War had recently begun in earnest. She implored her followers:

> Tell loudly and frequently to all your friends that you realize that it is unpatriotic to be fat while many thousands are starving . . . those not reducing at least one pound per week [should be] fined soundly and the proceeds given to the Red Cross.[44]

The thin "flapper" silhouette of the 1920s and the rise in popularity of Hollywood's "Golden Age" actresses of the 1930s[45] kept thinness an ever-present beauty goal for white American women. At the same time, the financial aftermath of the Depression, paired with the Dust Bowl's degradation of American food sources, made malnutrition a specter for many households. Recipes for casseroles, stews, and other low-cost, high-nutrition foods became the basis of bestselling cookbooks, and millions of Americans relied on public breadlines and soup kitchens to survive.[46] Fatness was portrayed in the media as a function of excessive wealth and privilege, often in the form of political cartoons depicting greedy politicians, bankers, and others blamed for the economic hardships of the day.[47]

During the Second World War, dieting again took on a patriotic flair. Food rationing made everyone reduce for the sake of soldiers who needed feeding on the front lines. Fats and sugar in particular were diverted. Fats went to make glycerin for explosives and sugar made sweets for soldiers in need of a quick energy boost for battle.[48] Scientists, prompted by the government, reported on how much "excess energy" resided in American fat, reporting that "a woman overweight by 40lbs. was to be accounted as hoarding 60lbs. of sugar in her excess flesh."[49] Fatness was beginning to be seen not only as "animalistic" and "gluttonous," like those pesky non-WASP immigrants, but "unpatriotic" as well—all resolutely un-American qualities.[50]

Note the singling out of female fat as the problem. Because most women were not on the front lines, they faced demands to do everything they could to aid their soldiers from home, including remaining as thin as possible. And as soldiers came home to their wives after combat, the men were often skinnier versions of themselves. Women's fertility once again arose as a national health concern and waistlines were monitored even more closely, as wives became mothers and re-populated postwar American society.

With the postwar baby boom, women, who had worked outside the home in place of men off to war, were returning to the home front.[51] Elite white, Anglo-Saxon Protestant families were leaving the cities, now overrun with non-WASPs, in favor of red-lined suburbs where they could create new, racially segregated communities. Suburban churches were built with plenty of Sunday School rooms to house their exponentially growing children's ministries. But there was a problem: many women didn't want to leave behind their independence and earning potential. And yet, here were the men, back from Europe and ready to take over the workforce once again.

Naomi Wolf[52] describes the tension of this time, with male advertisers and editors of women's magazines together creating a culture of WASP housewifery to restore the "proper" American social order.[53] They knew women would not just go back happily to the kitchens of yore. A new "benevolent sexism"[54] was born, one that kept women in their place but with the promise of fulfillment in the love of their husband-provider, the joy of their children, and—through capitalistic upward mobility—the delicious envy of their friends and neighbors.

To create a sense of fulfillment within the domestic sphere, advertising agents knew that women needed a new "professional" status within the home—home economics—and products of modernity, efficiency, cleanliness, and excellence that meant big money for the postwar economy:

> The marketers' reports described how to manipulate housewives into becoming insecure consumers of household products: "A transfer of guilt must be achieved," they said. "Capitalize . . . on 'guilt over hidden dirt.'" Stress the "therapeutic value" of baking, they suggested: "With X mix in the home, you will be a different woman." They urged giving the housewife "a sense of achievement" to compensate her for a task that was "endless" and "time-consuming." Give her, urged manufacturers, "specialized products for specialized tasks"; and "make housework a matter of knowledge and skill, rather than a matter of brawn and dull, unremitting effort." Identify your products with "spiritual rewards," an "almost religious feeling."[55]

The domestic goddess was born. And boy, did she diet.[56] The role of the WASP housewife was to remain "perfect" as a wife, mother, and domestic engineer. A very limited range of visual femininity was marketed to accompany that ideal—thin but curvy in the "right" places.[57] The full *ooh la la*. This is a shape very few women inhabit perfectly, at least not naturally, thus making diet and beauty products both indispensable and perpetual.

The white, upper- and middle-class body ideal of thinness thus moved from its origins as an Anglo-Saxon "racial" trait to part and parcel of the capitalist American Dream. Diet programs proliferated, moving from advertisements on the back pages of ladies' magazines into public life through TV shows. Stars like Donna Reed, that pinnacle of white domestic womanhood, and Lucille Ball went on diets as storylines in their television shows—despite their obvious thinness—all sponsored by commercials touting the latest diet fad. Group-based weight-loss communities like Weight Watchers sprang up, promising to help women stay motivated through friendship and accountability. These groups thrived as points of social connection—very much like churches themselves—full of new rituals of anti-fatness.

The countercultural movements in America during the 1960s had complicated effects on the 1950s idealism of the "traditional family." The Civil Rights and Black Power movements played out on television news alongside fears of "communism" and the Cold War. These were all threats that grew paranoia within elite white communities, which had made suburban fiefdoms around their WASP way of life and sought to keep them. The availability of women's birth control pills as of 1960 gave women the freedom to explore sexual pleasure for themselves unencumbered by fears of pregnancy, and the freedom to limit the number of babies in their family without their husband's permission. Women's dangerous natural power was out from under male control, and "bra-burning feminists" implored bored housewives to get in on the action. Once again, Naomi Wolf writes:

> Female fat is the subject of public passion, and women feel guilty about female fat, because we implicitly recognize that under the myth, women's bodies are not our own but society's, and that thinness is not a private aesthetic, but hunger a social concession exacted by the community. A cultural fixation on female thinness is not an obsession about female beauty but an obsession about female obedience.[58]

The Christian backlash against all of these threats to the "traditional family" and "traditional housewife" was swift. The Religious Right emerged as a powerful political entity and cultural force. Initially, they organized in 1969 as a loose conglomeration of likeminded conservative and fundamentalist Christian churches, individual evangelists and theologians, and politicians with one goal in mind: keeping Black-and-white segregation alive in American public schools.[59] They didn't even try to hide their racism at the beginning. But they soon realized that overt racism would only attract some "Christian" supporters. So, the movement's leaders took up the cause of "anti-abortion" and "family values" after the 1973 *Roe v. Wade* decision established abortion as a constitutionally protected right in the United States.[60] By focusing on abortion, the Religious Right, though WASP to its core, courted the support of conservative Catholics, whose ethical ties to the sanctity of all life made them particularly worried about abortion as a practice. Evangelist Francis Schaeffer was a central theologian in this movement to save the unborn, and he collaborated with a young pediatric surgeon, C. Everett Koop, to produce a series of films called *Whatever Happened to the Human Race?* depicting abortion, in the most graphic ways,[61] as a harbinger of greater (read: white) American moral decay.

C. Everett Koop, of course, would move from these auspicious beginnings to become Surgeon General through the 1980s under President Ronald Reagan and would famously declare America's first official "War on Fat" in 1994.[62] But he wasn't the only Christian concerned about waistlines. "Devotional fitness culture"[63] first emerged in the late 1960s—conspicuously beside feminism's rise in influence—and offered books, workshops, and full programs promising that people could pray themselves thin. This trend continues in earnest today.

Most Christian weight-loss efforts make explicit the connections that were brewing throughout American history between diet culture and the WASP way of life. They assert self-discipline as a moral virtue, promote the denial of all sinful "savage" appetites, and emphasize controlling the unruliness of the body, and women's bodies in particular. Beginning in the early twentieth century and continuing today, these values have been written onto American culture by white, middle- and upper-class Protestants whose positions of power in medical and political establishments created our current national health beliefs and values.[64] Sabrina Strings sums up the roots of America's diet culture:

> Never mind that prior to the late 1910s (elite white) women had been told overwhelmingly that they were too waifish, only to be told thereafter that they were too fat. This was despite the fact that a study of the U.S. Department of Agriculture on the weights of Americans showed relative stability between 1885 and 1955. The point was that these women needed to learn the scientific management of their bodies. Their own health, along

with that of their offspring, was the basis for the fitness of the race, and the nation.[65]

Sadly, our cultural anti-fat bias is one of America's great collective perpetuated traumas, passed down from generation to generation just like—and often because of—white supremacy. No one in this country is impervious to its biases. "Problematic fatness" has become part of our country's definition of itself, so much so that the exported caricature of "The Fat American" graces political comic strips from Topeka to Tripoli, a shorthand for excess, colonialism, and greed. And yet many fat Americans, like me, are just trying our best to live lives as happy and fulfilled as possible in light of the constant barrage of messages that denigrate us. Our best hope for fat liberation lies in greater education about the complexities of fatness and systems of fat oppression so that fat acceptance increases over time.

Readers who suspend their disbelief will find what critical fat researchers, fat cultural theorists, and fat activists have been saying for one hundred years now: fat people are not to blame for society's ills and owe no one an apology for our existence. Protests against "the culture of slimming" have been vociferous since at least the 1920s.[66] The "Fat Liberation Manifesto,"[67] written in 1973, spelled out the connections between capitalism, corporate greed, and the callous disregard for fat peoples' lives and wellbeing already clearly at work back then.[68] And it has only ever gotten worse.

Naomi Wolf adds this important postscript about the rise of diet culture in America, focusing on where it began—on limiting the power of women's bodies: "The great weight shift must be understood as one of the major historical developments of the century . . . Dieting is the most potent political sedative in women's history."[69]

CHAPTER 6:

THE POLARIZING FIGURE OF THE UNREPENTANT FAT WOMAN

Imagine with me a woman:

She takes up more space than anyone else in the room. She carries around 50-, 100-, 200-pounds more of flesh than other mere mortals, and navigates a world every day that was never meant to hold her. In this way, her strength is immense. She feels ocean-like ripples in every movement. She knows her difference is heavy on the minds of those around her, and she does not care. She knows her body intimately—its needs, fancies, and foibles—and gives it what it wants to the best of her ability. This is how she loves herself, how she honors the whole of her. She knows deeply that her creation is not a mistake and is still unfolding. She stands in awe rather than judgment. She knows her worth, knows her belovedness, her creatureliness, her finitude. She appreciates that this beautiful life will someday end, and savors both the ordinary and sublime. And what makes her life big is not her body but the way she lives in it. She is hazardous to any society that would have her shrink. She is dangerous, like the movement of the holy spirit across the surface of cultural status quo. She is a harbinger of change.

The image of an unrepentant fat woman is polarizing. To me, she is divine. This is to say that she knows God incarnate resides in the temple of her body, that she is the caretaker of that temple, and that she has great autonomy and authority. She can listen past the societal noise and hear God whispering from within that she is good and whole just as she is. To others, she is a woman betrayed by her biology, undone by her appetites. Perhaps the thought of God residing in fatness seems blasphemous. For those who understand fatness as a sin, the unrepentant fat woman is doomed to a hell of her own making.

The great sadness is that this is the hell to which diet culture calls us, counting our calories as dutifully as any rosary. Michelle M. Lelwica speaks of the "Religion of Thinness" at work in America, by which she means the commonly accepted practice of beliefs, commandments, rituals, myths, and even visual icons that together promise "salvation" in the form of ever-elusive bodily perfection and a blissful, superhuman longevity.[1]

The Religion of Thinness even has a liturgical year—bolstered by all forms of visual and written commercial media—which ticks along behind the backdrop of our society's cultural rhythms. The decadence of the fall and winter holidays leads to New Year's resolutions,[2] when the cabinets are purged of all offending foods and gyms are joined in earnest. This lasts a few weeks, perhaps, but not long enough. Superbowl Sunday splurges and Valentine's Day candy sales punctuate the winter grocery shelves. After one last binge on Mardi Gras, many are eager to recommit to their diets using the forty days of Lent to give up particularly tempting foods. The Easter candy is barely eaten before magazine covers remind us that swimsuit season is near. Summer fashions lead to further commitments toward reining our bodies in tight. When sweater weather finally arrives, we are glad for their bulky coverage, feeling freer to indulge ourselves with the comforting, decadent recipes of the fall and winter holidays. Rinse and repeat. This yearly cycle is so well known it barely registers to us as a phenomenon driven by consumerism and diet culture's simultaneous messages of consumption and restriction.

At the fringes of the Religion of Thinness are those deemed "out of control" and outside the bounds of presumed "health"—either too thin or too fat. These are the prophets of apocalypse. They are graphic warnings of a society unable to keep its people fed correctly,[3] imbalanced people either dramatically starving or over-consuming. Both insinuate by their very bodies that the supposed benevolence of our capitalist economy may not work for all people. But while both groups suffer stares, those who are considered ob*se, especially "morbidly" so, are society's Biggest Losers. Death fats.

Lesley Kinzel uses the expression "death fat" as the proper translation and cheeky "counter-euphemism" of the pathologized term for the largest fat bodies: "morbidly ob*se."[4] Though the term "morbidly" is slowly growing out of fashion in the medical industry, it was employed for decades and has added to anti-fat stigma and poor health outcomes for fat people. If you're told that you are death fat by your doctor (like I was when I was ten), why participate in your own body's care? You've already received a death sentence.

Kinzel and other fat activists now use the term "death fat" among themselves in defiance of a culture that imagines them doomed. Fats of any weight can defiantly claim death fat status, since all fat people, regardless of actual size, are imagined to be mortally endangered by their adipose tissue (plus, it just sounds super-duper goth). I say "imagined" because longitudinal studies have shown that fatness is synonymous neither with ill health nor exceedingly hasty death.[5] But once you're labeled death fat in this culture, you're understood to be a liability.

Kathleen LeBesco wryly calls us "Citizen Profane" and offers this critique of our country's collective anti-fat bias:

> The fat person makes the ultimate bad citizen in that
> she or he [or they] reveals the American Dream for what
> it is: a fabrication. If we put stock in a philosophy of
> limitless individual achievement through hard work and
> intelligence, then what is the fat person but a sign that we
> can't always get what we want?[6]

The monied meritocracy of middle-class white America is where fat hatred has gained its Pelotonic stride. This is the main audience to whom diet culture is marketed through media and over-the-fence word of mouth. Individual "freedom" to perform health and wellness becomes a social expectation,[7] just another way to keep up with the Jones's bodies. The work-hard-get-more-be-best neoliberal self-improvement pipeline is promised to work for all but the most abjectly idle—the lazy and the fat (who are usually considered one and the same).

US cultural imperialism does not care about different, collectivist visions of society, even though they form the ethnic origins of a growing majority of actual Americans. Different, equally valid visions of beauty, wellness, strength, gender, ability, and even health care exist among our non-white neighbors within this country and across the globe.[8] Within those communities, tangible *collective* support often surrounds those needing care; combined incomes provide for extended families' wellbeing; and in-group pride sustains long, even ancient histories of embodied knowing and rituals of health.[9] These challenge the *individualistic* health models, chronic body dissatisfaction, trust in modern medicine, and anti-fat bias that middle- and upper-class white Americans "know to be true."

The Religion of Thinness, that never-ending quest to colonize one's own indigenous shape, becomes diet culture's Manifest Destiny, writing external markers of white wellness onto already-good bodies. And all bodies are good bodies. But in America, it's the thin, the white, the young, the abled, and the rich body to whom we are all expected to bow in homage.

The Limits of the Body Positivity Movement

Scholar Andrea Elizabeth Shaw points to the "hyper-embodiment" of fat, Black women's bodies in American culture.[10] According to

Shaw, Black female embodiment provides an important critique of and alternative narrative to white hegemonic standards of beauty and wellness, which garners Black women a tremendous amount of societal stereotypes and disparagement.[11] Performers from Ma Rainey to Lizzo[12] gain notoriety not only for their tremendous talent, but for their "spectacle" as fat, Black women being unapologetically themselves.[13] Shaw understands the African Diaspora to be a cluster of cultures in which white Western ideals of slenderness as "beautiful and healthy" are not universally upheld, except perhaps where colonialism has taken hold.[14] This is what makes fat, Black women so "other" in white American society; they become, as Shaw writes, "the embodiment of disobedience."[15] And, truly, fat people of color have led the way since the beginning of fat activism, only to have their radical calls for "body liberation" eventually be shaped into modern-day consumerist "body positivity" at the hands of small-fat white women.

Fat writers of color are quick to point to the parallels throughout history (suffrage, civil rights, feminism) where white women coopted a radical message of inclusion only in order to fit *themselves* into the mainstream, leaving those still marginalized by race, class, and/or gender identity behind.[16] This assimilationist shift is seen in body positive spaces nowadays, which often focus on improving how fat women see themselves, rather than the more radical goal of trying to change the way society polices, judges, and treats all fat people.[17]

Similar to how Pride, which began as a counterculture symbol of radical queer liberation, has been coopted by corporations to sell their rainbow-colored products during the month of June, "body positivity" took the body liberation messages originating in the Fat Rights circles of the 1960s and repackaged them for the mostly small-fat, white female consumer.[18] Lane Bryant, The Body Shop, and Dove beauty products were examples of early adopters in the 1990s, using fatter women[19] in their commercials than the culture had seen before. Since the turn of the twenty-first century, the vastness of the internet has allowed fat women to make their own blogs, websites, and virtual communities, and many of these have focused on aspects of fat fashion (also known as "fatshion") and desirability. This has allowed fat women to self-style and promote a literally wider notion of beauty.

Fat representation, and especially fat self-representation, is liberative and important for society to see. As with other socially oppressed groups, representation matters. In that way, "body positivity" should be celebrated for its gains. Fashion and finding one's fearless self-expression can be political acts in themselves.[20] The critique comes, though, when primarily white, small-fat and medium-fat women are the only ones who benefit.

Some were eager to declare victory over anti-fat bias when Rihanna's *Savage X Fenty* lingerie line was launched up to a size 3XL (around a US size 24). No, Rihanna is just a smart businesswoman and decided to sell to a larger audience. If the goal is the opportunity to buy more things that fit and make me feel pretty, then body positivity is winning the day. But if the goal is true societal body liberation, then body positivity has stalled in its activism, distracted by shiny things. Virgie Tovar helpfully offers:

> As a straight, cisgender woman, I honestly understand the deep and hypnotic draw to assimilation. The closer you perceive your access to ideal citizenship to be, the harder it is to want something bigger, better. But fat activism told me that being accepted by the very people who made me feel less than human isn't enough. So why settle?[21]

Body positivity, at least as it's currently enacted, is mostly focused inward, toward how one feels about one's own fat body.[22]

It's a wonderful starting place for many fat people who just want to feel okay, even lovely, in their own skin. This is a worthy goal! But it cannot be the only goal. If I spend too much time focusing on loving myself then I will never get beyond that self-absorption.

Individualist notions of "self-love" is how body positivity, though packaged as a radical movement, often becomes the second side of the fat consumer's coin. "Heads" and it's diet culture asking you to buy another product to make yourself feel beautiful. "Tails" and it's body positivity asking you to buy another product to make yourself feel beautiful. Either way, individual consumerism wins and societal body liberation is put off for another day.

THE RECIPE BOX

I am a terrible cook. I can read a recipe but can't get the timing right to save my life. Should you come to my place for dinner, I would happily serve you appetizers at six o'clock, corn on the cob by 6:45, an overheated casserole around 7:30, and dessert at nine o'clock. All the fun of a progressive dinner without ever travelling to another home! Such is my culinary prowess.

My mother's orange plastic recipe box sits in a cabinet overlooking all of my cookery misdeeds. It is one of my most prized possessions. I know this because when I have made the mental checklist of things I would save in a raging house fire, Mama's recipe box ranks right after pets and purse and right before photo albums, a true pride of place in my tragedy-preparedness anxiety repertory.

The box is the luscious burnt sienna of 1960s color palettes. It provided the pop of kitchen color we needed against the avocado green Whirlpool refrigerator that somehow lasted our family more than forty years. The box is stuffed with recipes to the point that my fingers strain against their pulling. They are organized by tabs named Breads, Appetizers, Fish/Sea Foods, Sauces, Salads, Sandwiches, Soups/Stews, Vegetables, Desserts, Pies and Pastries (somehow distinct from desserts), and a surprisingly large section on Punch and Drinks. I remember Mama sitting down to type these recipes from various magazines or cookbooks onto thinly lined 3"x5" cards. She used her manual typewriter, a soft "shoot" whispered when she made a mistake and had to start all over again. Mama's neat cursive notes "cover with foil" and "can cut sugar in half" occasionally on the cards' margins, all indications of recipes tried over and over again, moving toward the mastery of personal taste.

To my childhood mind, my mother loved cooking. Why else would she spend her days in the kitchen putting three balanced meals together? Why make her own emulsified salad dressings or hand bread chicken thighs with corn flakes when she could instead buy the easier frozen chicken nuggets that I envied when I had dinner at friends' homes? We ate when my Papa got home from work in the evenings, but the kitchen would already smell delicious by my three o'clock arrival from school. I was welcome to sit on the counter and play sous chef to an unimportant detail like crushing the corn flakes, but otherwise I knew to stay out of her way. This was Mama's internal cooking choreography and her recipe box kept the time.

I understood that other families were not sitting down to traditional Southern "meat and threes" every evening like the ones prepared in my mom's kitchen. Her meals consisted of a main course (the "meat," though this could also mean a casserole) and corresponding three sides (usually two vegetables and a starch), plus a salad, a piece of bread with ample margarine, then a dessert. Thumbing through the recipe box now, I see the names of our weekly dinners and can taste by memory the Steak Italiano, Cashew Chicken Stir Fry, German Style Roast Beef, Quiche Lorraine, Taco Casserole, and French Delight dessert.[*] I thought I was a worldly eater, but it was only in the way someone who goes to Disney's Epcot might imagine themselves globally travelled.

Here's the typed-out totality of her Crab Meat *a la* King recipe, a favorite of Papa's that I remember as a frequent birthday dinner request:

> In a double boiler, empty two cans of crabmeat, then add three fourths stick of butter and small block of boxed cheese.[¥] Stir until cheese is melted. Serve over toasted English muffins. It's really gourmet—in fact, too good to be true.

---

[*] I am doubtful of the French origins of this dessert, given that its base is a mixture of instant chocolate pudding, cream cheese, and Cool Whip. But what do I know? Either way, it was *délicieux*.

[¥] Despite the brand evasion, the "small block of cheese" here is, of course, Velveeta, which also made its gooey appearance atop the Taco Casserole, Mama's signature chili, and even in her Christmas fudge.

It even reads like Donna Reed, right?

This concoction tasted delicious, I remember. It's a palatable metaphor of the white suburbs from which it originated: somehow both overly simple and overly processed, but not asking any questions.

I don't remember being taught this explicitly, but I knew from a very young age that I was meant to eat whatever was put on my plate, reaching for an additional helping of at least one dish to prove my appreciation for Mama's efforts. I loved her cooking, so this was no chore. All three of us (Mama, Papa, and me) were hearty eaters. We rarely had leftovers. But whatever remained would surely be incorporated into the next dinner somehow—mashed potatoes repurposed as latkes, bits of last night's pork loin in the green beans. Nothing would go to waste under Mama's home-economic eye.

Memories of my childhood dinners are impossibly idyllic. I am sure that I had a toddler's pickiness, a child's poor manners, and fidgety impatience. But the collective recollection is one of quintessential family rituals. Feeding us was my mother's performance of love, which we simultaneously appreciated and took for granted in the way that women who run households often are.

Our dinner table is where I learned how to use a fork and knife and to keep my elbows off the table, how to recite the Lord's Prayer and twenty-third Psalm from memory, at least most of the Apostles' Creed, and how to spell and count to a thousand. As an only child, I was in on the conversation, and I asked my parents questions fearlessly. I inquired about words I heard watching the nightly news with my Papa, and he would explain the Cold War in terms I pretended to understand. Somehow the punch line was always American exceptionalism.

We ate until everyone was full, I helped Mama clear the table, and we brought dessert into the den to eat in front of the TV before bedtime. Sleep. A new day, a new dinner to look forward to. I often asked Mama what was on the night's menu before leaving for school.

The ritual changed at some point. I remember it began with the absence of margarine on our table. And the solemn declaration that, as a family, we were all fat. Too fat for margarine.

Thus began a different sort of dinner ritual, one that centered not on the taste of our food nor on casual conversation but on calories and food groups, "exchanges" and smaller portions. I learned new things. I learned that my plate was not just a plate but a color-coded chart of how "good" or "bad" I was eating, and that I should cover two-thirds of it with green items for my meal to be healthy enough. I started spreading my peas out like soldiers one-by-one to stretch their amplitude and meet the protein section's front lines. My hands policed portions. I measured "one meat serving" by the flat of my small palm. My balled fist became one cup, my thumb two tablespoons. I was allowed a fingertip of "I Can't Believe It's Not Butter," which I could, in fact, believe was not butter. I chose to use this on my steamed vegetables since bread was no longer welcome. Mrs. Dash was our new dinner companion, a space always saved for her instead of Elijah.

Yet I continued to grow. My parents, too, remained bigger than they liked. I never noticed their size as a negative thing. I liked resting my head on Papa's big belly and listening to him snore as I watched *The Muppets*. Mama was the most glamorous person I knew. My body climbed and jumped and played just fine. I couldn't understand why we were all discontent with ourselves, at least at first. But it didn't take me long to learn the trick of body shame and to apply it liberally, like imagined margarine.

I recognize that I'm speaking of a privileged childhood, one with plenty of food to eat and love around the table regardless. Now that I'm grown, I know how much work it took for Mama to provide on this scale, the nutritional worries she carried in her shopping cart, the hope for my good future she stirred into every sauce.

I look closely into the tight organization of my mother's recipe box, past family favorites, to branded cards with names and tastes I cannot remember. They were clearly used several times but made no lasting impression. Weight Watchers cacciatore, described as "a 2-point sauce option to pair with 4oz. of the lean protein of your choice." Jenny Craig's "miraculous" eggless eggnog. Literally this is just sugar-free vanilla instant pudding mix watered down with skim milk to a drinkable consistency, then doused with cinnamon. Jenny, you need to find Jesus.

At some point, likely at bowling or bridge, Mama received the gift of a muffin recipe from a friend whose ballpoint scrawl promises, "You won't believe your taste buds! Better than chocolate chip cookies and only 60 calories!" Mama's three words, written in neat script across the card's corner, make me laugh out loud. They're as close as she could ever come to diet rebellion in red ink: "not worth it."

I wonder if she meant that the recipe wasn't very tasty. Or if the time involved to bake them wasn't worth their payoff. Perhaps the muffins themselves, only two tablespoons of batter each, were simply too small to justify those sixty precious calories. Maybe I'll make them to see if I can tell what she meant. No, I probably won't.

More likely I'll do what I did all through my childhood and trust she's steering me in the right direction. Then I'll probably go eat a chocolate chip cookie in her honor, savoring the flavors she loved so much, but also felt guilty for loving so much. And in this way, I'll honor her truest goal, which was always my happiness and wellbeing.

CHAPTER 7:

THE WAY WE UNDERSTAND "FAT" IS CULTURAL

(And if it's cultural, it's not unchangeable.)

"Fat" is a cultural concept. We write our beliefs and expectations, stereotypes and sins onto fat bodies in the United States, regardless of whether or not they're true. Because anti-fat hatred is as American as baseball (great exercise!) and apple pie (too many calories!).

But it wasn't always this way. As we've seen, at the turn of the twentieth century, the overarching fear in the United States was that women's bodies were growing too thin. Public health efforts were aimed at helping women put on weight, not lose it. There has been an incredible cultural shift in the policing of fat bodies over the past hundred and twenty years with the rise of US diet culture and the medicalized beauty-health-wellness industry. And this shift has, in turn, created even more fat people onto which we can pour our collective cultural disdain.[1] As a fat person, it's pretty disheartening to research this cultural shift. And, of course, it's even more difficult to live with the historical consequences of society's anti-fat bias each and every day.

Here's the good news: cultures can change over time. We know this to be true. The political and societal gains championed by those fighting oppressions as powerful as this country's racism, homophobia, and misogyny show how people united in a cause can slowly but surely effect that change. So, too, can anti-fatness, healthism, and sizeism be challenged. Just think of it. Fat could become understood as a neutral body type, not a problem to be fixed.[2] Infrastructure—mass transportation, chairs in public spaces, medical equipment—could be changed to fit and therefore welcome larger bodies. Media could stop making fat people out to be sad, sloppy, and under-sexed shells. Medicine could refocus its efforts away from adipose tissue itself and onto the complexities of diseases that affect everyone regardless of body size. Just imagine that: an end to fat hate in this country.

Free Your Mind and the Rest Will Follow

Oh, En Vogue. How right you were.[3]

Changing culture starts with changing oneself as an agent of that culture. It starts with peeling back the layers of what we believe to be true about ourselves and others and looking critically at why we think the way we do. Researcher Harriet Brown offers:

> When I give lectures on this subject, audiences often react with disbelief—at first. Our intellectual perspectives and emotional comfort zone around weight and body size have developed over years, and are reinforced constantly by much of what we see and hear. It takes time to understand things differently. And it can be scary to shift the paradigm; many of us have a lot invested in seeing things the way we've always seen them.[4]

The same can be said for white supremacy, capitalism, colonialism, or any number of systemic oppressions around us. And anti-fat bias is just another way to keep all but the most elite, white, rich, and thin bodies on the margins. While it may be hard to imagine a day without fat hate, one is definitely possible.

It starts with claiming fat identity. It starts with the chubsters and fat-bottomed girls, the big-boned and the fluffy, the sideshow fatties and the weight watchers all standing up as one great human mass and saying "enough." Enough of the self-hatred and body policing. Enough of the calorie counting that reduces the pleasure of food into equations of self-control. Enough with satiating our hungers in only the most ascetic, cardboard ways. Enough with the multi-billion-dollar marketing and media aimed at denigrating fat people as America's number one enemy. Enough of the myriad fat jokes, catcalls, and "health concern" comments that dot our daily landscape with emotional landmines. Enough of being told—explicitly and implicitly—that we are not beloved, not good, not whole until we lose enough of ourselves. Enough.

This is the greatest hurdle to fat acceptance in our culture: *the myth that fat bodies can magically become thin bodies if only they choose to do so.* It is the root of all the anti-fat bias and judgment that our society holds.[5] The idea that fatness is a mutable trait makes people judge fat folks as lazy and uncooperative in their own well-being. It makes those of us who are fat believe that we must be as weak-willed as they imagine us to be, piling on further shame and self-disgust. And it's a lie that has perpetuated tremendous harm.

So, let's interrogate that claim. Can fat people actually become thin people readily, with just a few better choices? And must we perform thinness to be of good health? Do our doctors actually want us to be healthy, or do they just want us to be thin? The answers are not what our medicalized diet culture would have you believe. If we can begin to dispel these myths, fat people and thin alike can stop the blame game. This is the only way our culture will change: if we start understanding fatness as a valid and permanent marker of personal identity.

The Myth of Sustained Weight Loss

I hope you're sitting down because I'm about to share a hard truth for those invested in weight-loss culture. The supermajority of fat people will remain fat people their whole lives. Eighty years of research shows that employing restrictive diets and exercise regimens for sustained weight loss works for only the tiniest fraction of people—think less than five percent.[6] Even then, the amount of weight kept off is minimal. Nutritional psychologist Traci Mann, who has spent twenty years leading the University of Minnesota eating research lab, analyzed all modern medical studies on long-term weight loss *ever written* and found that, on average, after two years had passed, the total average amount of sustained weight loss was just two pounds.[7]

Studies that claim the possibility of higher rates of long-term weight loss typically end their longitudinal tracking of dieters after a year or eighteen months, when some subjects are still under their original weight.[8] Thus, those studies can say, "Look! Long-term weight loss is possible!" even when they know that if their study lasted any longer, those same subjects would be back to their initial weight or, more likely, higher. Mann offers this description of weight-loss research:

> What you mean when you think of a diet "working" is not the same as what, say, the CEO of a diet company or an obesity researcher means. I suspect that for you, a diet works if you lose a lot of weight and keep it off . . . [for the CEO], a diet may work if people lose any weight at all for any length of time. And for obesity researchers, a diet might work if test subjects lose slightly more weight than people who are not dieting.[9]

Think of the money, time, life-altering restriction, and handwringing efforts people in the United States put into their dieting. We are not doing all of that for five percent of us to keep off just two measly pounds, people! I've put on that much weight after one good Thanksgiving meal, and I've lost that much just by having a cold.

While the vast majority of folks can lose some weight initially, even large amounts, they simply do not keep it off. This is the definition of "yo-yo dieting," otherwise known as "weight cycling,"[10] which Americans do as they move from one weight-loss plan to another, and then another, and then another, over time. A recent study of about 2,500 American dieters showed that they averaged 7.82 weight cycles over their lifetimes to date.[11] That is a lot of ups and downs, a lot of tried and failed diet plans. A lot of given-up New Year's resolutions.

Short-term weight loss through dieting is definitely possible, even likely,[12] but the long-term prognosis is, well, . . . I guess just don't throw out your fat jeans.[13]

The Myth of Poor Willpower

But the reason I can't keep off the pounds is due to my own poor willpower, right? Nope![14]

Just look at *The Biggest Loser* contestants over time. The National Institutes of Health took an interest in their long-term weight loss and invited them over for a study six years after the competition.[15] When surveyed, all but one of the fourteen participants had regained their weight, but this wasn't the most interesting finding. *Every single one of their metabolisms had changed*—slowed, in fact—making their bodies more susceptible to weight gain. This "metabolic adaptation" is thought to be a starvation response triggered by restrictive weight-loss measures like low-calorie diets and punishing exercise. When trying to exert control over fat bodies, those fat bodies tend to strike back. Or, rather, they try to adapt, protecting us from starvation.

Describing this phenomenon, which happens to everyday dieters just like reality television dieters, Michael Rosenbaum of Columbia University Medical Center offers:

> Your body is working to defend your energy stores—
> really your fat mass . . . When that fat mass is diminished

(either by eating less or exercising more) most of us respond by changes in brain circuitry that increase our tendency to eat and changes in neural and endocrine systems, and especially muscle, that make us more metabolically efficient—it costs fewer calories to do the same amount of work.[16]

So, even eating the same restricted-calorie diet they had before would be no match for the former contestants' slower metabolisms. Eventually, the weight comes back.

To be fair, most people don't lose weight at the speed and intensity of *The Biggest Loser* contestants. But, then again, as mentioned above, Traci Mann was tracking the usual slow-and-steady methods of dieting when she concluded *diets don't really work*.[17] Fat bodies will almost always reset to the same or higher weights, even if we keep our diet regimen going faithfully.

This is not only physically taxing but emotionally taxing, as well. Those who yo-yo diet report increased symptoms of depression and internalized weight stigma each time they regain their weight, which itself leads to all sorts of negative health behaviors.[18] Those of us who weight cycle seven or eight times across a lifetime still wind up fat, but in much worse shape than if we had just accepted our fatness to begin with.

Now, let's look at the inverse. What happens to a thin body that intentionally becomes fat? Ethan Sims at the University of Vermont did a study in which volunteers who had a medically "normal"[19] weight throughout their lifetimes ate up to 10,000 calories a day and increased their size by twenty to twenty-five percent, speeding up their metabolisms in the process. When the study ended and the subjects went back to their usual eating patterns, their bodies rapidly lost all the extra pounds, returning to their previous straight-sized weights within months and staying there into the future.[20]

The implication of all of this research is that genetic traits override[21] the behavioral interventions we attempt to engineer onto either fat or thin bodies. As part of her research into the effects of childhood weight stigma, Sondra Solovay found that, "a child from thin parents has a 3 to 7 percent chance of becoming fat. A child with one fat biological parent has a 40 percent chance of becoming fat. A child from two fat biological parents has an 80 percent chance of being fat."[22] Twin studies and adoption studies have backed this up further.[23] We try to outrun our genes at our own peril, given that the negative health and psychological effects of weight cycling throughout one's life are myriad, including potentially increased mortality.[24]

Said simply, thin bodies tend to stay thin, and fat bodies tend to stay fat. This used to be widely understood as a medical truth, before the age of diet culture intersected with medicine in the form of "ob*sity studies." The former American Academy of Medicine president, Woods Hutchinson, wrote in 1894, "[Fat] is really a most harmless, healthful, innocent tissue . . . the fat man tends to remain fat, and the thin woman to stay thin—and both in perfect health."[25] And both types of bodies correct to a personal "set point" weight if they eat consistently for their own body size, without restriction. Once we reach adulthood, if we do not consciously try to control our body size, and if diets have not already screwed up our eating patterns and metabolisms, our weight becomes "remarkably stable over time."[26] The fact that people who grow up thin tend to remain thinner, while those who grew up directly impacted by diet culture tend to be fatter, is evidence not of poor willpower but of how diets lead to higher weight over time.

All of these truths are well documented in the field of ob*sity studies. However, the idea that ob*sity is a normal genetic variant of the human body is not popular with those who sell weight-loss and wellness culture for a living. Much more important to their marketing is the idea that fat is not only unnatural, but dangerous.

From Neutral Body Type to Epidemic

The prevalence of anti-fat hate we consume as Americans is stag-gering.[27] Many historians of fat in US culture[28] show how disdain for fat bodies grew louder over the twentieth century, rising to its current apoplectic state starting with the invention of a national "War on Fat" in 1994.[29] The label "ob*sity epidemic," which began as a marketing ploy by diet industry leaders,[30] was taken up by the medical establishment, which welcomed research dollars from weight-loss companies to study fatness as a pathology, *a disease in itself*, rather than a body shape. As investigative journalist Alicia Mundy describes in her exposé of this era:

> The first rule in marketing is "create a demand" . . . So spokespeople for new organizations—groups such as the American Association for the Study of Obesity—with heavy funding from the drug industry and frequently companies selling fat-free products, upped the ante. Get people to perceive obesity as a disease itself, and you've laid the groundwork for selling pills and other medical aids, surgical procedures, and the like to cure it. People know cancer and diabetes are diseases and they require medicine. Get them to call obesity a disease, and you've changed the paradigm.[31]

With its rise to epidemic status, fatness became not only a personal issue but a widely discussed and demonized public issue as well, and a "moral panic" over fatness has since ensued.[32] Especially since the bar of who is counted as ob*se—which is to say, in the minds of doctors, *diseased*—continues to shift downward as the medical establishment realizes the insurance dollars available if millions more Americans are suddenly able to be treated for their fat.[33] Researchers then cite the suddenly rising numbers of

Americans defined as ob*se as further indication of a national health crisis *when doctors themselves were the very ones who lowered the standards to include smaller bodies in the ob*se category.*[34] It is true that Americans are getting fatter, but not exponentially, and there is little causal evidence to show this increased weight is itself responsible for any of the health risks or costs so often culturally associated with it.[35] And blaming fatness itself keeps researchers from studying structural factors—things like climate change, pesticide use, privatized water access, GMO's, environmental degradation, monied food lobbyists, antibiotic usage in factory farming, targeted food subsidies, preservatives and additives, and ethically suspect marketing—any of which may actually be causing some humans to become larger.

J. Eric Oliver, a professor of American political science and history at the University of Chicago, became interested in America's growing fatness and its political implications, and decided to research it for a book. In his own words:

> America, it seems, has a big, fat problem. Or at least this is what I thought when I started writing this book. Like many people, I, too, believed that America's growing weight was a genuine health quandary. Indeed, my initial plan for this book was to look at why we were gaining so much weight and what we could do to stop it. But then I started to examine the evidence and a funny thing happened—the more I read, the more I realized how misguided my initial assumptions about obesity were . . . What I came to realize was that, contrary to the conventional wisdom, obesity is not a problem because more than 60 percent of Americans weigh "too much." Nor is it a problem because hundreds of thousands are dying from being too fat. Nor is it a problem because it costs us hundreds of billions in healthcare

expenditures. Obesity is not a problem for any of these reasons *because none of them are true.*[36]

And yet, those are the headlines we hear in a nation "at war" with fat,[37] and thus a culture swimming in anti-fat bias. In her study *Fat Shame: Stigma and the Fat Body in American Culture,* Amy Erdman Farrell offers, "if we are at war, then fat must be the enemy. And, by definition, we seek to destroy enemies in a war, not to engage in diplomatic missions of understanding or research."[38] This focus on fat eradication at all costs has, in turn, continued to line the weight-loss industry's coffers, which was exactly the original goal of the invention of the "ob*sity epidemic" in the first place.

CHAPTER 8:

AN UNHOLY TRINITY: THE DIET, BEAUTY, AND MEDICAL INDUSTRIES

The American market for thinness has supply-and-demanded ob*sity into a physical and moral problem that then can only be resolved in capitalistic ways. It's a perfect cycle that exists only so long as fatness is hated. Which it increasingly is. And, thus, the weight-loss industry has exploded in value over the past fifty years, especially as it has repackaged itself and changed with the times.

Sonya Renee Taylor, fat activist author and founder of TheBodyIsNotAnApology.com, speaks of the "global Body-Shame Profit Complex"[1] as a synonym for the way big industries (food production, medical wellness, beauty, fashion, and media) come together to infuse consumers with body shame while simultaneously providing the very products that, for the low-low price of $49.99 per month, promise a cure from said shame. Julie Guthman, a professor of social sciences at University of California, Santa Cruz, calls out the inordinate attention given to ob*sity as the "political economy of bulimia," with capitalism both the feeder and the purger of modern fatness.[2]

In 2019, the weight-loss industry was worth seventy-eight billion dollars. Its worth declined by an historic twenty-five percent in 2020 as many wellness clinics and gyms shuttered because of the Covid-19 pandemic. Yet in 2021, the weight-loss industry recovered nearly all of that loss, pulling in 72.6 billion dollars[3] as many people tried to lose their pandemic pounds (referred to jokingly by some as their "Covid-19"). The forecast for

2022 is once again industry growth, with the market expected to swell by at least 3.6 percent.[4]

The weight-loss industry's monetary value is pieced together by many interlocking diet-related companies, including medical weight-loss programs (such as bariatric surgeries, hospital inpatient and outpatient weight-loss programs), gyms and health clubs, apps and streaming services (such as Noom and Peloton), diet meal replacement companies (such as SlimFast and Nutrisystem), commercial diet center social programs (such as Weight Watchers and Jenny Craig), the retail diet food industry (like Lean Cuisine), diet and wellness self-help books (like keto, Atkins, and South Beach diets), exercise DVDs, streaming video, and weight-loss and appetite suppressant pharmaceuticals (fun fact: these are known as "nutraceuticals" because they constitute such a large part of the pharmaceutical industry). Each year, market research companies compile huge reports analyzing the diet industry and all its facets. They sell tomes of this data for thousands of dollars back to both industry leaders and upstarts looking to tap into the highly lucrative weight-loss market. Market research companies promise that their data reports uncover the kinds of consumer trends that will allow these weight-loss companies to maximize their profits.

For example, the 2021 *The U.S. Weight Loss & Diet Control Market* report compiled by Marketdata, LLC, was sold for $2,195. It covered the "consumer clean eating & high protein trend," the "shift to do-it-yourself methods" by dieters during the 2020 pandemic, suggested how diet companies can reach Millennials in a section called "The Millennials Dilemma," and targeted profiles of dieters by "budget, starting weight, preferred diet plan location, type food desired, previous diet plans used, readiness, exercise plan desired, % needing psychological support, [and] % with special food needs."[5] They wrapped up their report with a meta-analysis of all trends and concluding recommendations for the 2021 "diet season." These included the use of softer, less diet-y words focusing on bodily strength, health and wellness, and disease prevention rather than on weight loss. "Anti-diet dieting" is the new trend, it seems, but why?

"Clean eating"[6] has been championed over the past decade by celebrity chefs, food journalists, and Instagram influencers simultaneously touting the dangers of the processed food industry to both bodies and the environment. The ketogenic diet, or keto, has been the prevailing diet trend during these same years, dovetailing exacting nutrition rules of "clean," unprocessed foods with strict rituals of intermittent fasting. The other big weight-loss trend of the decade has been communal, push-your-body-to-its-limits exercise clubs like CrossFit. Millions feel they've benefitted from these regimens, and that's fine. Part of fat liberation is the desire for people to be free to use their bodies in whatever way they personally choose. I'm delighted for those who can do a hundred burpees in a row. That's surely an extraordinary feat of strength and endurance. And maybe a breakfast of two boiled eggs, four almonds, and eight green beans, followed by eighteen hours of fasting, and then a twenty-one-ounce porterhouse steak with extra butter is satisfying. If so, may the ketones be with you! But apparently the sheen of that particular regimented health-and-wellness coin, the one where bodies are so tightly controlled and monitored, is wearing off. I can almost hear the thud of a million kettlebells dropping to the ground at once. Folks are tired. And cake is delicious.

Just take a look at the most recent bestselling diet publications. They have names like *Clean Enough, Do What Feels Good*, and *Eat What You Love*. In their review, *Publishers Weekly* says, "what emerges from these books is an expanded definition of healthy: one that makes room for indulgences, shortcuts, backslides—even love handles."[7] Caroline Dooner, a popular yoga and fitness coach turned blogger, recently published *The F*ck It Diet: Eating Should be Easy*,[8] which takes direct aim at the diet industry's historic marketing plan of yo-yo diet weight cycling as damaging to one's health (#truth). Dooner, who is not fat, writes of her own weight-loss history:

> Even the times when dieting "worked" and I was actually skinny, it was never, ever enough. I didn't *feel* skinny, or worthy, or confident. And the moments that I *did* feel skinny? I was mostly *panicked* that the skinniness wouldn't last, and that made me even more obsessed with dieting . . . but . . . *diets don't even work.* The way we try to exert control over our bodies is biologically flawed and set up to fail from the start.[9]

Clean eating, exhaustive exercise, and other forms of extreme body control are facing a backlash, even from the fit-and-healthy crowd. They see how eating disorders have risen over the past decade,[10] especially "orthorexia," which is defined as "an obsession with consuming only foods that are pure and perfect."[11] The Covid-19 pandemic further exacerbated America's fixation on "health and wellness." Researchers found that the stress of enduring a deadly pandemic provoked many people struggling with disordered eating to deepen their overly regimented patterns of food consumption and exercise as a means of thwarting a generalized fear of sickness and death.[12] This was reinforced by the US government's narrative of "personal responsibility" for one's pandemic health, which media was happy to spread widely.[13]

So, all of these trends (critique of too-clean eating, fear of illness, exhaustion at super self-controlled dieting efforts, personal responsibility narratives) are digested and metabolized by the weight-loss industry, and out they excrete new, more palatable diets, which are not marketed as diets at all. I'm looking at you, Noom.

A mobile weight-loss plan disguised as "health coaching," Noom has grown by leaps and bounds since its arrival on the weight-loss scene, with more than fifty million downloads.[14] Its revenue grew exponentially from the start, accelerating even faster during the Covid-19 pandemic. Noom made twelve million dollars in 2017, sixty-one million in 2018, 237 million in 2019,[15] 400 million in 2020,[16] and was expected to generate 600 million dollars in revenue in 2021,[17] making it one of the fastest-growing private companies in the United States.[18] Noom's marketing includes the true admission that diets don't actually work, but it follows this right up by promising "but this one will" and touting a sixteen-week plan to reach one's weight-loss goals.[19] This is a perfectly pivoted dieting platform.

The fifty-six-year-old brand Weight Watchers, realizing the same translate-dieting-into-wellness trends all the way back in 2019, rebranded itself as "WW" and added the alliterative tagline, "Wellness that Works."[20] They also launched "Kurbo," another "health coaching" app aimed at children eight to seventeen years old, which widened their market to fat kids and their freaked-out parents.[21] (Beware, parents, because the lasting effects of dieting on children of any age are dangerous to both their bodies and self-esteem.[22])

Professor of American studies and gender studies Amy Erdman Farrell likens the US diet industry to the country's military-industrial complex, especially in light of the pervasive "War on Fat" language. She writes of President Eisenhower's warning of a massive, self-perpetuating military establishment:

> [This military establishment is] enmeshed with a large arms industry whose point becomes more about maintaining itself than about the ultimate purpose of the government—to maintain peace. Maintaining the giant military-industrial complex actually precludes the push for peace, as it requires that our nation maintain a constant state of war . . . Just as the purpose of the

military-industrial complex is to maintain itself, not to seek peace, the purpose of the diet-industrial complex is to keep people dieting (or choosing surgery, diet pills, or membership in clubs) rather than to seek health.[23]

No matter how companies rebrand, repackage, and reframe, it's all just the same giant commercialized diet-industrial-complex aimed at making sure you and I hate and fear fatness. And no matter what "lifestyle change" program we ascribe to, our money, time, and personal effort goes to further feed that industry.

This is not new information. Researchers and public health officials, psychologists and epidemiologists, physicians and lawyers, philosophers and historians have long pointed to the capitalistic gains bound up in our public health concerns about ob*sity. It's just that the monied voices of media, medicine, and weight-loss marketing are much, much louder. When fat people are maligned by society to the point of being seen as a disease, confirmation bias fuels what we "know to be true" about fatness,[24] even when there is ample evidence to the contrary.

Confirmation bias is the tendency we have as humans to interpret any new information we learn through the lens of what we already believe to be true. The direct marketing of anti-fatness during the twentieth century until today has created a culture in the United States in which fatness is a hated trait for most people, whether on their own bodies or on the bodies of others. Weight-based bias and the accompanying stigma placed on fat people are quite literally deadly problems.[25] Prejudiced doctors spend less time with their fat patients and miss important physical cues for serious illnesses because of their hyper-focus on weight.[26] Fat people fear going to the doctor because they know they will experience weight stigma, regardless of what brought them in for their visit, and thus avoid positive health behaviors like regular mammograms,

Pap smears, colonoscopies, and even basic checkups.[27] All of this leads to fat people frequently being diagnosed with diseases later and at higher stages of development, when the effects of an illness are harder to reverse. "Recommending different treatments for patients with the same condition based on their weight is unethical and a form of malpractice," says Dr. Joan Chrisler of Connecticut College. "Research has shown that doctors repeatedly advise weight loss for fat patients while recommending CAT scans, blood work or physical therapy for other, average weight patients."[28]

Doctors' substandard treatment of fat patients begs the question. Is it that fatness is itself unhealthy, or does weight-based bias in the medical industry keep fat people from lifesaving intervention and care? Though the latter is likely truer,[29] any research that is funded by industrial weight-loss interests or conducted by the very doctors who run "weight-loss clinics" is always going to say it's the former. And that, folks, is confirmation bias at its most killer.

If all people enact confirmation bias when engaging the world, then that includes the very doctors, journalists, and researchers who study and further interpret fatness back into the mainstream of American culture. While we hope for scientific objectivity, the idea that researchers are somehow superhumans, immune to cultural influence or personal proclivities, is as nonsensical as believing one's pastor to be immune from sin. This is a naive and dangerous belief that is simply not true. The orthodoxy of "scientific truth" obscures human fallacies and failures all the time,[30] just as the clergy collar obscures plenty of faults and foibles. Studies of confirmation bias within media[31] and medicine are fascinating,[32] and give a glimpse into why we don't hear the full truth about fat in our doctor's offices. Those who have already decided fatness is fundamentally problematic are in charge of its research and care. Implicit bias has the loudest microphone on fatness in this country, even when the narrative borne out by ob*sity research itself is hardly monolithic.

There is, for example, ample research that shows body corpulence can actually *help* people survive certain chronic diseases, and that most folks deemed medically "overweight" and "ob*se" are no more likely to die early than their thinner counterparts.[33] Do you know what ob*sity researchers call this growing group of studies, which do not fit the "fat equals unhealthy" paradigm that underlies the majority of public health efforts? They call it the "ob*sity paradox,"[34] a name that itself belies bias. They must name these studies a "paradox" because anything positive—or even just not overtly negative—said about fatness undermines their anti-fat research and worldview. One cannot assume that scientists are unbiased in their research efforts or that they are immune to the anti-fat culture in which they function daily.[35]

The research conducted by several prominent scholars of ob*sity shows how the medical industry has caused more harm than good by its incessant weight-loss interventions.[36] James S. Puterbaugh wryly calls his fellow American ob*sity researchers "The Emperor's Tailors"[37] because their diet, exercise, and surgical health interventions actually contribute to the very negative health outcomes they are supposedly trying to prevent.[38] His study of the medical literature on diet, exercise, and weight loss from 1879 through 2009 shows how, in his words, "the profession basically backed into the problem [of ob*sity] with treatments based on unexamined assumptions,"[39] recycling individual methods known not to work and eschewing societal changes that might lead to health improvements for thin and fat people alike. But, for a new paradigm to emerge today, the medical industry's implicit anti-fat bias would need to be addressed, and the commercialized weight-loss industry would need to be disentangled from both the research and treatment of ob*sity. A Herculean task, though not impossible because, as we have seen, cultural bias around human differences can change over time.

Harvard University's Implicit Association Test (IAT) has been available publicly since 1998 and is a valid and reliable measure for people's implicit bias around a number of human differences, including skin tone, gender, age, sexuality, disability, and weight.[40] The test is free and open to researchers and the general public, and thus has become a well-used source for tracking the development of cultural biases over time. While measures of explicit bias can be confounded by peoples' unwillingness to admit they are biased, the IAT uses the indirect measure of a person's response time to pictures of certain people as a measure of the implicit opinions they hold about the people represented in the pictures. In a review of 4.4 million tests administered from 2007 to 2016, researchers showed improvements in American cultural implicit bias of sexual orientation, race, and skin tone, while age and disability attitudes stayed neutral over the decade.[41]

The only measure in the study to *rise* in implicit bias over these nine years was weight-based stigma, which rose by a whopping forty percent in the face stimuli test,[42] prompting the researchers to posit that there must have been a widespread cultural effect in the United States that made respondents' attitudes about body weight more negative over the decade. A look at just the 2016 IAT statistics showed a full eighty-one percent of test takers had anti-fat and pro-thin bias.[43] That points to a pretty widespread cultural trend. Again, kudos to the diet-industrial complex for its impeccable marketing schemes.

But it wasn't just commercial weight-loss companies driving home anti-fat stigma during the nine years between 2007 and 2016. Fat activist and author Aubrey Gordon points to the Obama presidency, out of which came a series of local and national health initiatives "asserting the personal responsibility of adults, children, and their parents to become and remain thin."[44] I still think Michelle Obama is an actual goddess, but her "health and wellness" focus in the White House[45] was yet another reboot of the decades-long presidential "fitness-as-citizenship test" that has indicated to generations of school children and their parents which bodies (thin, fit, abled bodies) are most ideally American.[46] The weight stigma arising in kids of all sizes from such national "wellness" initiatives lasts their entire lifetimes[47] and can have dramatically negative effects on their overall health.[48]

The Ill-Health Effects of Dieting: The Minnesota Starvation Experiment

During the Second World War, physiologist Ancel Keys and psychologist Josef Brozek conducted a now famous scientific study nicknamed the Minnesota Starvation Experiment.[49] It's a classic both because it is so widely known and because its likes have not been seen since. A longitudinal study of starvation probably couldn't be carried out today, given modern ethical restrictions on using human subjects in research.[50]

The study's goal was to help the military understand how many calories soldiers needed on the front lines, the effects of starvation on their bodies and minds, and the best way to recuperate those who returned from the war undernourished. They chose thirty-six male volunteers—conscientious objectors who were glad to put their bodies on the line for scientific experimentation but not for fighting—and for three months fed them the 3,200 calories a day that was considered a normal amount of food for a healthy adult male.[51] The men worked and walked for exercise, staying on-campus in lab dorms so their behaviors and health could be closely tracked. After their initial three months of monitoring, the men's diets were cut in half to 1,600 calories per day for the next six months. For the purposes of this experiment, 1,600 calories was considered "semi-starvation," and we should pause here to remember that this is the same number of calories the FDA has recommended daily to fight ob*sity.[52] A full 1,600 calories may even sound like a splurge to those of us who have been on "cleanse" and "quick loss" diets that can total as few as 800 to 1,000 calories per day.

Well, on only 1,600 calories of daily food intake, these guys began to experience both physical and psychological symptoms, which gradually increased over time. The men had been chosen from a wide subject pool expressly because of their physical strength and psychological wellbeing. Keys and Brozek wanted to study the "best of the best" possible soldiers. And for the first three months, they were reported to be in good spirits as they worked and engaged with one another. But once introduced to semi-starvation, the men quickly began to change.

First, they reported a loss of energy, followed by a general sense of apathy about their lives and a lack of clarity in thinking. Their sex drives and senses of humor began to wane. They became irritable and their care for their body hygiene lapsed. The men experienced depression, restlessness, mood swings, and anxiety—some to the point of self-harm.[53] Every one of them became obsessed with food. They would think about food all day, fantasize about their next meal, read cookbooks, sneak in food behind researchers' backs, get irritable if they weren't fed on schedule, and enact rituals of eating slowly or drinking in-between bites to make their mealtimes longer.[54] What the men were allowed—unlimited water, coffee, and chewing gum—became preoccupations, sometimes even addictions. Some men drank fifteen cups of coffee; others chewed forty packs of gum per day.[55] Several simply broke their starvation with hidden binges before starting the regimen up once again, reporting shame over their loss of self-control.[56] One of the stranger symptoms had to do with the men's body dysmorphia around weight loss. They did not perceive their own bodies growing smaller, but instead began seeing other people's bodies as too fat.[57]

Even with all of this, the physical symptoms of starvation were perhaps even worse than the psychological. The men's bodies atrophied in both muscle and fat and their heart rates fluctuated. They lacked coordination and experienced soreness in their muscles; some saw edema (water retention) in their joints and their hair began falling out. They did not have the energy to exercise, so they became more sedentary overall; they avoided their chores in favor of rest and sleep; and their metabolisms slowed by forty percent.[58]

Unfortunately, all was not well when these men began their recuperation, which was also monitored by the researchers. Keys began increasing subjects' daily intake of food slowly—in three different groups to see which method of starvation recovery went best. One group received 400 calories extra per day, the second 800 additional calories, and the third were restored the full 1,600 additional calories that returned them to their pre-starvation levels of feeding. For all three groups of men, though, these additional calories were not enough. Even those fully restored to their original 3,200 calories per day stayed ravenous, and while on average they consumed 5,000 calories per day, a few consumed upward of 10,000.[59] Many of the men had lasting psychological effects, including a phantom sense of hunger that could not be satisfied for months—even years—after the experiment had concluded.[60]

I mentioned that the Keys study was one of a kind because it can't really be replicated under modern-day scientific norms of human subject research. You just can't sequester subjects for eighteen months and starve them in the name of science. However, this *is* an era where 1,600 calories is a typical daily goal for many dieters. Researchers can, therefore, study the negative effects of restrictive dieting, and they certainly have.

Sondra Solovay offers her summary of these studies:

Weight-reduction diets have been tied to all of the Keys's symptoms as well as others including: decreased growth in children, decreased mental performance (equivalent in degree to consumption of two alcoholic beverages), gallstones, cardiac disorders, fainting, psychological trauma from weight-loss failure, anemia, stroke, nausea, gouty arthritis, poor nutrition, aches and abdominal pain, elevated uric acid levels, delayed healing and scar development, changes in liver function, cardiac problems, and death.[61]

It is not only unfair but dangerous for fat people—or people of any size—to be expected to choose a form of starvation, with these subsequent medical and psychological ills, as a means of performing American diet culture. It also speaks loudly to the level of anti-fat bias in our medical industry that, knowing all of these potential effects, doctors still readily prescribe diets to "cure ob*sity." It's cruel, and it has effed up millions of us. As I read through the Keys experiment, I saw myself in many of the reported symptoms. Perhaps, if you have dieted, you do too. Thankfully, researchers are beginning to see these links between the illnesses that get blamed on fatness and dieting itself.[62]

An alternative exists. We can agree to no longer restrict our caloric intake in any way, eating what we want when we want to, trusting our cues of hunger.[63] If that sounds like an impossible decadence, it is diet culture talking. Some nutritionists and doctors are pointing to unrestricted eating as one way to save ourselves from the harms that dieting does to our minds and bodies.[64] And people are not necessarily gaining weight. But neither are they losing it.

And so, a question remains. *Even if it is healthier to do so*, are we willing to embrace our fat, rather than dying to lose it?

CHAPTER 9:

BIG FAT TRUTHS ABOUT OB*SITY

People who are physically fat can be healthy.[1] There. I said it. Thankfully, lots of actual ob*sity and public health researchers have said it, as well.[2] In fact, studies show that anywhere from one-third to three-quarters of those deemed ob*se are actually completely metabolically healthy.[3] Meanwhile, about twenty-five percent of thin folks are metabolically unhealthy.[4]

Now, if this is difficult to believe, like it initially was for me, please know that this is because of how ingrained diet culture is in our everyday lives. And because of how much money is poured into making cultural anti-fatness stay that way.[5] It takes a veritable worldview shift to begin to unravel the tangle of anti-fat messages trying to sell "lifestyle changes" from the big, fat truth that "overweight" bodies are not necessarily any more unhealthy or undisciplined than their thin counterparts, and that restrictive dieting often causes more medical harm than good.[6]

Even the research that is paid for by the diet companies themselves says this.[7] Doctors know it, too.[8] Harriet Brown, a scholar who studies the weight-loss industry, offers:

> Doctors know the holy trinity of ob*sity treatments—diet,
> exercise, and medication—don't work. They know yo-yo
> dieting is linked to heart disease, insulin resistance [type
> 2 diabetes], higher blood pressure, inflammation, and,
> ironically, long-term weight gain. Still, they push the same
> ineffective treatments, insisting they'll make you not just
> thinner but healthier.[9]

Hold up, wait just a second. Doesn't that list of ailments she mentioned sound a lot like the ones doctors usually ascribe to fat itself? Fat is considered unhealthy because it leads to [*go back and read the list in Harriet Brown's quote*]. Uncanny overlap, right?

We don't even have to look back to the Minnesota Starvation Experiment to know that restrictive diets are harmful, either. A growing amount of recent research shows that dieting,[10] especially from a young age,[11] can cause health issues like these more reliably than living in a higher-weight body over the course of a lifetime does.[12] And weight loss, when achieved, doesn't actually lead to improved health in and of itself.[13] Just because one becomes thinner does not mean one becomes healthier, despite all the messaging we receive to the contrary.

It is also not true that fat people, on the whole, eat more or exercise less than the general population. Americans of all sizes eat poorly and exercise less than medical doctors would like us to! Only ten percent of Americans eat the "proper nutritional balance," and only twenty percent meet the weekly exercise guidelines of thirty minutes a day, five days a week.[14] And yet, the thin person who does not perform these health behaviors is not imagined to be in danger when they purchase processed foods, sit on the couch for Netflix marathons, and snack on Cheetos. It's just that their metabolisms and genetic makeup allow them to do these things without gaining a large amount of adipose tissue. "Thin privilege" is the ability to pass as "healthy" and thereby fit into society without weight discrimination.[15] This means greater systemic access to resources like health care, insurance, employment, social desirability, and even airline seats.[16] One does not have to actually feel thin, or even good about their body, to gain access to thin privilege; it's simply the proximity to the visual "healthy ideal" that grants it.[17]

Fat people, on the other hand, are universally thought to be endangered by their weight, and their personal choices are blamed regardless of their actual health behaviors. Fat activist Lesley Kinzel speaks of the #TwoWholeCakes phenomenon, birthed when an online troll accused her and other fat people of *literally* eating two whole cakes each and every day. She says:

> The phrase "two whole cakes" is appealing because it is ridiculous. It evokes the kind of insatiable appetite and gratuitous pleasure seeking that our culture so erroneously assigns to fat people. It suggests a total loss of self-control, the danger that—as Marianne Kirby has put it—fat people will "eat the whole world." It is also very funny. It's useful to zero in on negative stereotypes and show how preposterous they are.[18]

When we examine our beliefs about fatness—our own and others'—are we compassionate, understanding that our size is mostly genetic, and that our health is not causally tied to our body weight? Or do we imagine two whole cakes?

Is Ob*sity Research Slowly Catching On?

A 2015 study in the journal *Critical Reviews in Food Science and Nutrition,* helmed by a team of twenty-four public health and medical researchers, conducted a meta-analysis of nineteen widely held assumptions about fatness and weight loss.[19] What they found was that each of these popular anti-fat narratives lacked sufficient empirical evidence. And yet, they noted, these inaccurate beliefs still shape our medical decisions and public health policies. These unsubstantiated theories inform the use of severe ob*sity treatments that threaten lives. And they feed the all-important cultural narrative that fatness itself must be eradicated. Speaking to the entire medical health enterprise, their study concludes:

In the current [ob*sity] research environment, we often believe things to be true and demonstrated when they are not true or not proven . . . This begs the question, why? Perhaps, some ideas seem so sensible that we never stop to ask for the data. Psychologists are well acquainted with the mere exposure effect, which states that the more we are exposed to something, the more we come to like and believe it. Is it possible that if we are simply repetitiously exposed to discussion of obesity with the commonly used, vague words of implicated and linked that we will come to believe that the proposition has been proven? Conceivably, some ideas are so precious to us that we cannot bear to let them go despite evidence to the contrary. Or, we allow ourselves to be satisfied with weak data. Of course, there is also the more malign possibility that some people are deliberately distorting the available evidence to match their preconceived notions.[20]

Five years later, in 2020, thirty-six ob*sity and public health researchers, most of them holding credentials within the weight-loss field itself, signed a joint statement that called for ending both public and medicalized stigma associated with ob*sity, once and for all.[21] Researchers unaffiliated with weight-loss interventions have decried the effects of anti-fat bias for years. But this new statement was different because it came from within the very "ob*sity studies" field that creates and upholds medicalized weight-based stigma. These ob*sity researchers had changed their minds and, in their article, now called weight stigma a "pervasive, global issue."[22]

The thirty-six signers first reviewed and summarized the literature on the negative health effects of weight-based stigma before declaring:

The notion that the causes of overweight and obesity depend on individuals' faults, such as laziness and gluttony, stems from the assumption that body weight is entirely under volitional control. This assumption and many of its corollaries are now at odds with a definitive body of biological and clinical evidence developed over the last few decades.[23]

They used their research to dispel some common misconceptions about fat people, including: that body weight is a simple equation of calories in, calories out (it's not); that fatness is caused by eating too much and not moving enough (not usually); and that diets and exercise work to make ob*se people thin (nope). They called for primary care doctors, policymakers, researchers, the media, and the general public to stop equating fatness with laziness, personal choice, or ignorance, as none of these things are borne out by their research.

In yet another countercultural study, a research team of epidemiologists led by Paul Campos of the University of Colorado evaluated four central claims of the ob*sity studies field: the ob*sity epidemic affects nearly every country worldwide; higher-weight individuals die sooner than "normal" weight individuals; the data linking fat to ill health are "well established and incontrovertible"; and significant long-term weight loss is possible and improves health.[24] Their findings were nope, nope, nope, and nope. They concluded (emphasis mine):

Given the limited scientific evidence for any of these claims, we suggest that *the current rhetoric about an obesity-driven health crisis is being driven more by cultural and political factors than by any threat increasing body weight may pose to public health.*[25]

When ob*sity researchers themselves start saying these things, maybe things will start to change. It's a hopeful thought. But there's such a long way to go.

They Don't Treat Us Because They Don't Study Us

People over a certain body weight cannot donate their bodies to science for study after their death,[26] nor their organs for transplant.[27] This is supposedly because of the practical concern of not being able to move or store larger bodies. Many cadaver tables in use today are made for bodies that weigh less than 200 pounds. But this seems to me a pretty flimsy excuse for not studying in depth the majority body type of Americans. More likely at issue is the fact that the presence of fat makes a body more difficult to dissect, even described by some doctors as "unpleasant."[28] But again that excuse is a poor one. Doctors using the "yuck factor" doesn't seem like a valid response when proctologists exist. This is more likely further evidence of anti-fat bias at work in medicine.[29]

Pharmaceutical companies do not routinely test their medications on "the ob*se" as a distinct group of people, even though we are such a large percentage of the population. This means that if I'm prescribed medicine, doctors are pretttttty sure I'll be okay if I use it. But trials do not exist for bodies like mine, and fat people often trade horror stories of being over- or under-dosed by doctors doing their best pharmaceutical guesswork when the research just isn't there.

A great example of this danger came at the expense of Aidy Bryant's character "Annie" from the Hulu TV show *Shrill*. Originally conceived by fat author Lindy West,[30] *Shrill* has received lots of praise for the way it accurately describes being a young fat white woman in America today.[31] Early in the series, Annie becomes pregnant after taking the emergency contraceptive "Plan B," otherwise known as the "morning after pill." When she returns to her pharmacist she is shocked to learn that the pill doesn't work for women above 175 pounds.

Often fat women learn the effects of their bodies remaining unstudied-yet-over-medicalized too late. A tumor goes undiagnosed, or mounting symptoms are ignored, all because a doctor sees and attempts to treat their fatness first as the ultimate health priority. There are harrowing stories of fat people[32] not being believed when they know something to be wrong in their bodies, then winding up with higher-stage cancers and more advanced disease as a result.[33] This kind of fat stigma from doctors, not our adipose tissue itself, keeps fat people from pursuing wellness measures. Fat people do not want to continually be blamed, ridiculed, or disbelieved,[34] and so they also sometimes avoid seeking health care altogether as a result.

This is familiar territory for me. I was once prescribed a liquid diet when I went in to see my doctor for an earache. Another time I was told by a gynecologist that she was "a little worried" that the steel table stirrups might not be strong enough to fully hold the weight of my legs, so could I please hold them up myself as much as possible during my exam. I will say, it is very difficult to hold one's fat legs in a strange out-and-yet-also-sort-of-up angle for the full length of a pelvic exam. Every time I lightly rested my feet on the cups of the stirrups, trying not to bring the whole apparatus crashing down under my somehow enormously-powerful legs, I imagined my doctor rolling her eyes at my lack of core strength. I couldn't actually see her face because she was wearing a mask and also staring directly into my vagina. Then, at one point near the end, as she was trying to extract the speculum, she had the audacity to tell me I was "clenching." Ahem. She had no idea how much.

When medical instruments don't accommodate fat people and doctors are not encouraged to study fat bodies, this limits the range of care fat people receive. And when we do receive care, our presenting symptoms are often ignored in favor of prescribing weight loss as a cure for every ill. Some doctors have dropped the pretense entirely, simply not agreeing to treat patients above a certain size because they are considered too risky and/ or uncompliant.[35] This anti-fat bias directly contributes to poor healthcare for fat people, and medical structural weight stigma becomes a self-fulfilling prophesy. As fat activist author Ragen Chastain writes, "the problem is that [doctors with anti-fat bias] are practicing stereotypes instead of medicine."[36]

It's as if the medical establishment has made up its mind on fatness and is content with its current bias. Perhaps that's because it's so financially lucrative.

There's Big Business in Ending Big Bodies

We believe fat is terrible because it must be that way to perpetuate the weight-loss industry. If people weren't concerned with their size, there would be no one to download Noom! The trick is that the very people selling us on weight-loss products and bariatric surgeries are often the same ones funding anti-ob*sity research. These studies, then, start from a place of anti-fat bias and seek to further inform the medical and cultural pro-weight-loss narrative.

Journalist Harriet Brown notes, "I've been told by numerous researchers that the easiest way to get a study funded now is to include the word 'obesity' in the proposal. Even better, cite 'childhood obesity.'"[37] There is huge cultural interest in eradicating fat. Lobbyists funded by diet drug and weight-loss companies crowd government hallways to ensure the "War on Ob*sity" remains a well-funded enterprise. The science behind weight-loss imperatives thus becomes muddied by special interests aimed at human waistlines.

There is an unethical financial codependence between medical research on ob*sity and many facets of the diet industry.[38] The messages we receive that fatness is a "disease" from our doctors and mainstream media are based on research funded by the commercial and medical weight-loss programs and diet drug companies themselves.[39] Doctors who personally profit as the heads of bariatric and weight-loss clinics are tapped to serve as our nation's "ob*sity experts" while simultaneously being paid to sit on the boards of commercial weight-loss programs. The National Institutes of Health (NIH), World Health Organization (WHO), and other organizations that write government public health policies, employ these same ob*sity experts, who, in turn and unsurprisingly, recommend their own products as the exact "lifestyle change" necessary to eradicate fat. This is the "tail wagging the dog," as they say.

Nutritionist Traci Mann talks about how, all the way back in the 1990s, when anti-fat bias first became substantiated into the "ob*sity epidemic" by then Surgeon General C. Everett Koop, the government began to scrutinize the weight-loss industry's research and practices. The Federal Trade Commission (FTC) asked representatives from the various commercial and medical diet programs to come together and produce the guidelines for advertising weight-loss programs. Yes, you read that correctly. *They asked the diet industry to self-regulate its marketing efforts.* Unsurprisingly, this clearly-biased group came back insisting that weight-loss marketing guidelines should not need to offer proof of effectiveness at all. Mann describes their decision:

> They said they would not offer data on the efficacy of their diets in the short term or the long term, or even the number of people who completed their programs after starting them, which are pretty much the exact facts potential customers would want to know. The representatives of the diet programs gave amazingly unconvincing reasons for why they should not have to provide this information. First,

they argued that it was too costly and difficult to collect such information, even though many of them already had the information on hand. Second, they said, dieters don't need this information because they have had lots of experience with diets and are already very knowledgeable about them. Their third argument, though, was the most illuminating. They said, as recorded in the FTC report, "Dieters will be discouraged if they are provided with realistic outcome data." This was nothing less than an admission that their programs were not effective. The diet companies won the battle—they still do not have to disclose any of this information in their ads. But their unwillingness to report on whether their diets are effective makes it clear that they do not have much confidence in their diets, and they don't want you to know it.[40]

The diet industry is self-regulated, and this is ethically thorny at best. Weight-loss programs know that their products hurt, or sometimes even kill,[41] fat people, but are allowed to go forward with their use under the faulty logic that it's better for a person to die from their product than the perceived "ill health effects" of fat. What a terrible dehumanization of fat people who should be allowed to live lives full of dignity at all sizes.

The diet industry testified that "dieters will be discouraged if they are provided with realistic outcome data."[42] Yes, yes, we would be. The only thing keeping the self-regulated diet industry in business is cultural anti-fatness. Without it, perhaps we'd stop trying to lose weight and start trying to live happily as the fat people we were born to be. This is what fat activists mean when they remind us that our culture doesn't have to be full of anti-fat bias. With more education and critical insights into diet culture, things might start to change.

THE PARABLE OF THE TWO KNEES

She is a marathoner whose knees gave out at thirty-seven after a young adulthood of cross-country running. She had four different surgeries before the age of forty-five. All of these were covered by her health insurance, and she runs proudly still at fifty, titanium joints now absorbing every stride.

She was never much of an athlete. High school tennis, college intramural softball. Since then, she's mainly found her body moving to keep up with her young children—two boys of rambunctious age. When she slipped and fell on ice a few winters back, she banged up her knee, but kept making snow angels despite the pain, as mothers often do. Months later, when things still weren't right, she went to her doctor, explaining her initial fall. The doctor prescribed a seventy-five-pound weight-loss regimen, starting with a liquid diet for two months. "That, or you could get bariatric surgery," he offered. She protested, reminding him that, before her icy fall, her joints were working perfectly. "Yes, but if you hadn't been so overweight, the fall would not have damaged your knee so much," was his quick retort. The doctor was clear that there was nothing he could do. Insurance wouldn't cover joint surgery for someone her size, anyway, though it would readily cover laparoscopic stomach stapling. She would simply *have* to lose weight before her knee could be fixed. Three years later, she is still trying to lose the seventy-five pounds necessary to fix her knee, the pain of which now keeps her from playing too much with her boys.

Which woman is worthy of healthcare?

CHAPTER 10:

THE QUESTION OF "HEALTH"

Can I ask you a personal question? If you had the choice between your body being a perfectly proportioned example of toned, socially desirable thinness and yet unhealthy, or 400 pounds and yet healthy, which would you choose? And why? Please take a moment. I will eat this cracker and play with my dog Henry for a minute while you do.

This is ultimately a trick question for fat activists, because "health"[1] is both elusive to define and problematic as a universal goal. Its use as an ideal subjugates as "other" anyone who naturally falls outside of the boundaries of health and wellness. By centering "health," we are always going to leave out, for example, superfat and infinifat folks, most of the aged and elderly, and those who are chronically disabled either mentally or physically in some way. Many of us in this country will never get to say we're "healthy" for a whole host of reasons. And those that can will not likely stay "healthy" throughout their lives.

Arguments for any singular standard of wellness—even if eventually widened to welcome small-fat bodies—implicitly presumes a social hierarchy born of proximity to "health." Millions of people never achieve "health" and still live meaningful lives just as they are.[2] Here is where the work of fat studies intersects with the work of disability studies.[3] Both undergird activism that seeks the decoupling of human dignity from capitalistic understandings of individual ability and productivity toward more socialized policies of *collective* care and *societal* wellness—the kind of true "healing" Jesus embodied in his own ministry (which we will discuss further in chapter 14).

American culture makes "health" a primary goal of its citizenry because a person's wellness presumably translates into their productivity as a worker and, thereby, their ability to be a consumer.[4] (Hello, capitalism!) I hear this sentiment repeated in the anti-fat hate messages of both mainline and social media alllllll the time, its shorthand being some version of the phrase, "fat people are a drain on society."[5]

First of all, this statement is inaccurate. If fat people cost the healthcare system "more" than the average person (and this is a big "if," given that most ob*sity statistics are greatly inflated),[6] it's not actual fatness that's to blame when weight loss is our only prescribed cure no matter what ails us, and weight loss has been shown to be physically harmful. In other words, this is a cyclical problem. There's a fatphobic medical system diagnosing adipose tissue as a disease and then prescribing weight-loss interventions known to be harmful as its only "cure." This medical myopia is not accidental, but represents a well-orchestrated effort[7] to make ob*sity into a health epidemic so that those who benefit financially can continue to do so.[8]

A quick aside: a word should be said here about researching fat bodies. You'll remember my mentioning in chapter 9 that fat bodies are under-researched. They're not used in most pharmaceutical trials, not practiced on in medical school, and not allowed to donate their bodies to science for deep dives into their unique physiology. This lack of study leads to substandard care. All of this is true. So why am I claiming here that ob*sity is *over-researched*? Great question![9]

Remember the definition of ob*sity found in chapter 2. Ob*sity is a medicalized word based on the underlying assumption that fatness is a self-caused disease that must be eradicated. There are tons of research studies on ob*sity. There's big money in trying to figure out the "cause of ob*sity" so that it can be stopped, in linking fat to underlying health risks (by correlation, not causation, mind you),[10] and in studying the efficacy of various means of weight loss. All of these studies are based on the idea that my fat body is a problem as it is, even with no health issues. Because, to ob*sity studies researchers, my fat *itself* is the issue, a "disease" regardless of its actual effects. The assumption is that *of course* I want to lose weight, when what I really want to do is be treated equally to my thin peers, dignified in the fat body I have and will always have.

No ob*sity study is meant to help me live life in this good, fat body of mine. Alternative research on *fat and fat people* exists, but it's not nearly as funded as ob*sity research, and sometimes it must link itself to weight-loss interests to even garner funding. But more fat-neutral medical research could help systematize proper prescription amounts for larger bodies. It would foster the invention and retooling of medical instruments to serve a wider range of body sizes, and it would help doctors learn how to treat and operate on fat people, rather than just prescribing us weight loss. All of these things would help de-stigmatize fatness and increase positive health outcomes for fat people. I dedicate this paragraph to the amazing Ellen Maud Bennett, a vivacious sixty-four-year-old Nova Scotian who was diagnosed with inoperable cancer after years of doctors missing her symptoms and prescribing weight loss, instead. Her obituary called them out, saying:

> A final message Ellen wanted to share was about the fat shaming she endured from the medical profession. Over the past few years of feeling unwell she sought out medical intervention and no one offered any support or suggestions beyond weight loss. Ellen's dying wish was that women of size make her death matter by advocating strongly for their health and not accepting that fat is the only relevant health issue. Please remember Ellen when you next read a great

book, go to a play or buy a small object of stunning beauty. We've lost a remarkable woman.[11]

Our question about fat research vs. ob*sity research answered, let's go back to the prevalent idea that fat people are a "drain on society." This invites the dangerous corollary of naming other oppressed groups as similar "drains." We hear echoes of this when politicians talk disparagingly about families on welfare or undocumented immigrants. Lawmakers seek to defund social programs like food stamps while also refusing to raise the minimum wage so a family might live above the poverty line. People are told to "work harder" so as not to be a drain on the system, even while that system stays firmly stacked against them. This is verbatim diet culture logic when you think about it.

Such "drain on society" thinking becomes even more deadly[12] in the hands of those who would use violence to scapegoat a particular populace in the name of reducing their supposed negative influence on society. In the United States, eugenics campaigns led to the forced sterilization of people with disabilities and minoritized, particularly Black and Indigenous, women well into the twenty-first century.[13] This was a medically sanctioned form of genocide, and it (or something like it) could absolutely happen again.

Fat studies author Kathleen LeBesco notes the eugenic nature of the fight to eradicate fat, which often takes on the language of human genetic improvement.[14] The worrisome thought for LeBesco, and for anyone claiming fat identity, is that if, for example, a "fat gene"[15] could be isolated and eradicated, society's rampant fat hate would almost certainly lead to the widespread use of this therapy. One study showed that eleven percent of people surveyed would abort a child if they knew in advance it would be predisposed to fatness.[16] That survey took place in 1994, and our society has become far more anti-fat since. I wonder what the results would be if it were re-run now.

As long as American culture continues in lockstep formation against fat people, and the narrative of ob*sity's great collective drain on our society intensifies,[17] fat activists rightfully ask whether governmentally enforced diets or bariatric surgeries might one day greet us in the name of "the social good." Difficult to imagine? I hope so. But the moment we turn a certain type of people into an epidemic, a disease, something to be eradicated, we're heading in that direction.[18]

This is what makes the task of claiming fat identity such urgent work! It's literally necessary to my survival as a fat person, and to the survival of anyone who loves their body, respects all bodies, and wants to see body liberation rooted in universal human dignity rather than some dystopian capitalistic form of "health" performance.

Say it with me. All people should be allowed to exist, and even provided the opportunity to thrive, without cultural shame—fat people, sick people, disabled people, and people marginalized in any other ways. Say it again. Say it until you believe it. Say it until you believe it applies even to your own fat body, or to the body of the fattest person you've ever seen.

The "Healthy" Consumer

Fat activist Charlotte Cooper speaks of capitalism's influence on notions of "health," saying:

> Where there is no safety net of welfare, people face
> great pressure to be fit for the marketplace, to present
> themselves as competitively employable, to be winners.
> Fat people represent failed citizens within this frame,
> the slow, unwell, undisciplined, unemployable losers
> in the race of life whose only chance of betterment is by
> participating within neoliberal health regimes.[19]

Here Cooper points to the preference in neoliberal politics for everything to be the fault of the individual in order to limit the responsibility of a government to care for its citizens.

The citizen-as-consumer-of-health is a correlate to the concept of "individual responsibility." The thinking goes like this: a productive worker will be able to earn enough money to make themselves well through their individual choices and buying power. Consumerism allows us to buy ourselves "healthy," to perform our "best selves" back to society and earn its respect. But the sneakiest part of the neoliberal capitalist health-wellness-beauty industry is that there's always more to buy, so long as "health" remains an undefinable, elusive goal!

Even if a person is "healthy," their public performance is never, ever enough. Are you skinny? You need also to be toned. Are you toned? Then how about some plastic surgery to stay looking young? What does it mean when "looking young and healthy" becomes the goal and our bodies naturally shift over time? According to the beauty and diet industry, lithe, pubescent bodies represent the apex of wellness.[20] Health's blue ribbon. With that goal, the aging body, the fat body, and the disabled body don't stand a chance.

It's no wonder we pull out our pocketbooks to buy whatever they sell us. The cooperative health-wellness-beauty industries can always invent and repackage their programs and products to get our populace *even* fitter, *even* stronger, and *even* more culturally "beautiful." There is always something more to buy because, no matter how hard we try, we cannot reach perfection. Sigh. Diet culture is one of the most obvious forms of neoliberal consumerism that we have, and yet everyone just sees "fat" as the problem.

Think about the chronically ill person unable to hold down a job, or the infinifat who can be legally discriminated against by hiring employers in forty-nine of fifty states.[21] It's likely that neither of these people can afford costly health insurance without a subsidized workplace plan, nor would they be coverable within the private insurance market due to their pre-existing conditions. Their only chance at access to health care comes from socialized medicine; this is what "health care for all" is supposed to mean, and why it is so necessary. Even those of us who are "healthy" today, whatever that means, may very well become "unhealthy" tomorrow. Those of us who fight for fat inclusion must not center "health" as the most desirable trait, but instead value all bodies—especially those that are marginalized and told (in myriad implicit and explicit ways) that they are therefore disposable citizens.

"Healthism"

Any time we focus on "health," instead of inherent human dignity and collective societal care, we push "unhealthy" people aside, and we reinforce neoliberal ideas of personal responsibility and consumerism as means of moving up this country's citizenship hierarchy. And by posing the uncomfortable question at the start of this chapter—would you rather be thin and unhealthy or fat and healthy—I have fallen into that old, exceedingly unhelpful trap of defining health in a singular, individualistic way.

However, this book is meant mainly for readers just encountering the truth of diet culture for the first time, who have not yet embraced fat identity nor fat activism. These are the folks who need a question that puts the idea of "fat and healthy" in stark contrast with "thin and unhealthy." It helps get to the root of how we think about "health" in the first place.

What do we mean when we say we want to be "healthy"? Do we really mean "metabolic health" or are we mostly looking to physically perform health by looking thin or fit? Do we want to feel "as good as we can for as long as we can"? Well, that can be done in a fat body, too! And when we leave our fat bodies alone and don't try to manipulate their size, they tend to be metabolically healthier.

But if the thought of being really fat but otherwise healthy is anathema, then we must ask ourselves why. It usually doesn't take much personal inquiry to notice how our concerns with "health" intersect with our anti-fat bias.

Here's the thing: increasing positive health behaviors (things like drinking water, moving our bodies, and eating plenty of nutritiously and emotionally satisfying foods) reaps health benefits, *even if they don't cause any weight loss at all.*[22] Professor Amy Erdman Farrell recounts nutritionist Lindo Bacon's two-year study of "weight loss" vs. "health-behavior change" groups over time.[23] While most participants within the dieting group initially lost some weight, by two years into the study, half of them had dropped out and most regained their weight. Typical diet results, nothing new. The second group was coached to listen to their bodies' hunger cues, stop counting calories and instead eat a variety of nutritious foods; move in fun and fulfilling ways; and, importantly, participate in a *fat acceptance* study group.

The second group was not cajoled toward health with promises of a "brand new body" but instead invited to feel good in the fat bodies they already inhabited. Their health measures, like blood pressure and cholesterol, as well as overall self-esteem, improved significantly over the two-year period and not one person dropped out of the study.[24] The lessons learned from their study led Lindo Bacon to write their popular book *Health at Every Size.*[25] Known by its acronym "HAES," this set of fat-neutral health principles originated before Bacon; fat activist circles of the 1970s had already long been calling out diet culture and anti-fatness as medical harms.[26] "Health at Every Size" has now been trademarked by the Association for Size Diversity and Health (ASDAH), a network of size-inclusive practitioners and fat activists,[27] and it is growing in influence as an alternative to the usual harmful anti-fat narratives of diet culture that permeate the medical field and wider society.[28]

By all medical counts, those in Lindo Bacon's second study group became "healthier" than the first group did, but they also lost no weight. And health researchers have found that, without the promise of losing weight, people are unmotivated to increase their health behaviors. Most people are willing to adapt their diets and increase their exercise *only* if it means "they will look better,"[29] which is to say in this tremendously anti-fat culture of ours, "thinner."

I'm going to invite you to come over here and sit with me and Henry-dog on this couch so we can pause for just a moment to think about this. Let's consider all the messaging we receive about how terrible fat is for our health.[30] People's disgust for their own and others' fat is couched in concerns of what they are "doing to their bodies" with added girth. America's costly "War on Ob*sity," with billions of funding dollars pushed toward public health measures that encourage restrictive dieting across one's lifespan, is supposedly aimed at its citizenry being "healthier." Doctors prescribe life-threatening bariatric surgeries to make their patients more "healthy," not just thinner, right?

But could it be that what truly concerns us nowadays is not "health" at all, but rather the perception of health, with thinness as its visual proxy? Could it be that the medical industry has become so intertwined with the diet industry that being thin is now understood as the only actual way to be healthy?

Amy Erdman Farrell, in her book *Fat Shame: Stigma and the Fat Body in American Culture,* speaks to this, saying: "Experts acknowledge that modest changes in diet and exercise will improve a patient's health but will not necessarily make the patient *look* healthier—that is, thinner. In a culture permeated by fat stigma, a thinner body provides the illusion of health."[31] She is speaking here of the counterintuitive effects of "healthism,"[32] and how it has, over the past century, slowly overridden "health" as the main medical and cultural concern around fatness in America.[33]

Healthism was first described by Robert Crawford in the early 1980s as a preoccupation with wellness that, at its core, understands personal health to be under one's own individual responsibility and control.[34] Healthism's most dangerous corollary belief is that any person can "achieve" personal health if they try hard enough to do so, thus moralizing those who can't achieve health as lacking in willpower or tenacity. Thus, "healthist" bias arises toward those who aren't—or don't look to be—healthy.

But health is both relative and mitigated by a host of internal and external factors. Genetic differences (like predisposition to certain diseases) and societal differences (like socioeconomic status) play extraordinarily large roles in one's overall health. Racism, sexism, anti-fatness, and other systemic oppressions limit health, as well.[35] These societal conditions are known as "social determinants of health" for the way they influence a person's physical wellness, and are gaining traction in the medical research thanks, in large part, to the rise in critical race, fat, and disability research since the 2010s.

Yet healthism's effect has been strong on both the medical industry and wider society over the past four decades, posing a great danger to public health. Blaming individuals who are unwell for their own ill health reduces the public's will to prioritize systemic public health solutions like eradicating poverty. Also, by elevating health as the ultimate moral value above all others, healthism further privatizes the struggle for systemic human thriving. For example, why create walkable sidewalks and pedestrian infrastructure in areas of lower socioeconomic status when everyone can download a cheap workout app on their phones? This "no excuses" line of healthist reasoning forgets that not everyone has a viable electronic device with adequate bandwidth or the free time to prioritize working out.

Health is always easier to achieve for the privileged, yet healthism suggests an egalitarianism that simply does not exist.

Crawford concludes:

> To the extent that healthism shapes popular beliefs,
> we will continue to have a non-political, and therefore,
> ultimately ineffective conception and strategy of health
> promotion. Further, by elevating health to a super
> value, a metaphor for all that is good in life, healthism
> reinforces the privatization of the struggle for generalized
> well-being.[36]

Healthist bias is at work when people see me and make assumptions based on my large size. The stranger who yells, "eat a salad" while I'm walking through my local subway station does not know my eating patterns. He doesn't know that the reason I should, in fact, go and "eat a salad" is probably because I skipped lunch altogether.[37] His healthist concern is not actually about my health at all. It's about him. My fat offends him, and it becomes an imagined shorthand in his mind for a host of gluttonous behaviors. Or perhaps, because he spends a certain amount of money, time, and energy on his own body to look a certain way, he assumes I should share those values, and that, if I did, surely, I wouldn't be so terribly fat. But my body is different from his. We have different genetics, social locations, and hormones. There's very little likelihood that my body would react the same way to his regimen, and I do not owe him one damn minute on an elliptical machine. Healthism is at work any time someone else tries to decide my health for me—either by stereotyping what it is or implying what it should be.

Healthism has arisen alongside the capitalistic medical diet industry, now so ubiquitous an underlying system that it goes unchecked for the ways it hurts people—not just fat people, but anyone on the margins. Anti-fat weight-loss culture is yet another example of American "bootstrap" culture in which those who are oppressed are told they must be the source of their own salvation, rather than count on the changes to society that might fully include them and help them thrive. Any time individual responsibility is judged paramount over ending corporate greed, our capitalistic system has won again.

Fat activists emphasize that there are systems of oppression surrounding health norms and the research that upholds these norms. As mentioned, oppressions like racism, economic poverty, and other social determinants of health affect public wellness in profound ways.[38] Yet American society's weight-biased narrative largely ignores these realities, always turning back to the supposed sin of fatness and an individual's responsibility for their own health.[39] Meanwhile, the oppressive systems in which fat people (and all people) must live and move go unchecked.

This is true even with increasing evidence that the stress and trauma of living as a marginalized person in society often *itself* causes significant negative health outcomes.[40] Researchers are now studying the link between the chronic stress[41] of living in an "othered" body and higher cortisol production, which leads to heart disease, weight gain (particularly in the midsection), slower metabolism, insulin resistance (type 2 diabetes), depression, anxiety, and eating disorders, among other things.[42] Note the similarity between that list of ailments and those blamed on fatness.

In short, weight stigma itself can cause many of the illnesses[43] doctors so easily attribute to excess fat. So, it is reasonable to argue that abolishing the stigma rather than the weight would make sense. As one ob*sity studies research team from York University in Toronto recently noted:

Conformity to dominant models of the obesity and health relationship by health sciences researchers, public health workers, and the media lead to activities that rather than promoting health, actually threaten it . . . we call for an end to seeing obesity as a significant health issue.[44]

They are calling on the culture to change.

THE CARROT

My nutritionist moved to the edge of her chair and held her palms out flat, offering me a choice. She smiled and asked with the breathy, wide-eyed excitement of a kindergarten teacher, "Do *YOU* know the *DIFFERENCE* between *THESE* two foods?"

"That one is a carrot, and that one is an Oreo cookie," I said flatly. I was eleven and had never felt so patronized. Of course, I knew the difference between these two foods. The differences were obvious. One was a vegetable and one was a cookie. One was good in salads and one was good literally any time.

I was a fat kid, but I had eaten far more carrots than Oreos in my lifetime. By the time I was trotted off to the nutritionist by a concerned pediatrician, "junk food" hadn't been allowed in my house for years. Yet, like she had done through the entirety of our weekly sessions to date, my nutritionist was once again making false assumptions about my diet. Otherwise, how could she explain the bulk of me?

And so, we played this ridiculous comparison game for about fifteen minutes each time we met. She would hold out pictures of two foods, and I was to pick the "good" choice. Her goal was that I would learn how to make these same choices in the real world. Three Cheetos or a bunch of grapes? A chicken breast or a cheeseburger? A chocolate shake or a cool glass of ice water? One of these is nutritious while the other is not, and therefore should never, ever be eaten. This was an exercise in black-or-white, good-or-bad dichotomous thinking about food.

She also measured the speed of my choices—the faster, the better. To her mind, she was instilling in me the cat-like reflexes necessary to stave off the onslaught of complex carbohydrates just waiting to jump me around every corner. "Don't think! Just choose!"

she cheered me on. *Become one with the flashcards; become one with the game.*

I just couldn't do it. The carrot/Oreo comparison was so ridiculously, maddeningly condescending. This whole game was, really, and yet I stayed because as a kid I didn't feel I had the agency to leave. And I stayed because I desperately wanted to lose weight. I wanted to be the same size as my friends and wanted all the approval that I was sure would come with a thinner frame. I was tired of my weight being the focus of every meal, every bite preapproved for consumption, then marked down in a food diary. And I was terrified of the imminent death promised to me over and over by doctors and weight-loss professionals, a premonition that they swore would come true if I couldn't learn to choose the carrot and deny myself the Oreo.

She tried to convince me that, chewing it slowly for a good deal of time, the sweetness of a carrot would actually eventually taste *better* to me than the Oreo did. Because carrots were, and I quote, "the dessert of the vegetable kingdom!" Oh, how I hated this woman.

She implored, "No! *HOW* are they *DIFFERENT?*"

"The carrot is good and nutritious and the Oreo is bad empty calories," I acquiesced while reminding myself it was rude to roll my eyes at an adult.

"GOOD!" she smiled and reached into her desk drawer. She handed me a plastic baggie with a large carrot inside. I stared like the dumb fat kid she thought I was. "Here! You can have it as a treat! Let's chew it 100 times before swallowing and see if we can taste the sweetness!" The "we" always meant "me," so, with a loud crunch, I took a comically huge bite.

100 . . . 99 . . . 98 . . . I used every chew as an opportunity for silence, a respite from the condescension. And while that carrot never tasted like dessert, I told her that it did.

SECTION THREE:

IMAGINING FAT CHURCH

"The safest places I know
(the ones where everyone is queer
and everyone is nonviolent
and socialist and anti-racist
and everyone has learned how to listen
how to open their hearts
how to be very gentle with themselves
and each other)
are
still
fatphobic
as
f*ck."

—@megelison on Twitter, 8/ 10/ 18, 10:27PM

CHAPTER 11:

DISBELIEF IS A STARTING PLACE

You know when you read something so farfetched that you do a double take? You think "no, that couldn't be," and then start doing your research to figure out if it's true?

Take, for example, the final resting place of Fredric Baur, the inventor of the iconic cylindrical Pringles potato chip can. He was cremated and, per his request, his ashes were buried—you guessed it—inside of a Pringles can. Original flavor, of course. Don't believe me? Look it up.

Or the fact that a man once ate an airplane. Every bit of it. It took Michel Lotito, a French entertainer who became famous for eating indigestible objects, two years to finish the Cessna 150. To be fair, it was just a four-seater. Don't believe me? Look it up.

The longest recorded amount of time between two sets of twins being born was 87 days.

The tongue is the strongest muscle in our bodies.

And female kangaroos have not one, not two, but three vaginas. Don't believe me? Look it up.

I offer you these hard-to-imagine-yet-true facts because I'm guessing a great many readers for whom this is new information may be swimming in "that-can't-be-true-ness" at this point in the book, which is a *completely fine* place to start the work of ending anti-fat bias through the gospel of body liberation. The story of how fat turned into the "ob*sity epidemic" (cue the scary music) is full of facts that are strange to most of us who have been enculturated to hate fatness. Anyone encountering this information for the first time might think, "No, that couldn't be." I felt the same way at one point.

It couldn't be that weight loss and diet drug company executives lobbied US government officials in the 1990s to manufacture a "War on Fat" that would validate the use of their products. But it's true. The "ob*sity epidemic" began as a marketing ploy to rewrite fatness as a disease so mortally dangerous that companies could sell weight-loss drugs that knowingly killed some of their users. If their pills were deadly, they needed fatness to be understood as even deadlier in order to be legally absolved from blame.[1]

It couldn't be that health institutions as trusted as the Center for Disease Control and World Health Organization allowed inaccurate statistics about "mortality from ob*sity" to be reported and circulate widely in order to maintain funding for their research efforts. And though these statistics have been debunked repeatedly, because they were once said by these institutions, they continue to be cited in the medical literature and media as fact.[2]

It couldn't be that ob*sity wasn't actually designated as a disease until 2013, and that this decision was made by the American Medical Association so that bariatric surgeons and other weight-loss doctors could gain access to insurance money for their services. Since then, BMI standards have continued to be lowered, making smaller and smaller patients "ob*se," which therefore makes them eligible to have these expensive and dangerous medical interventions using insurance.[3]

It couldn't be that when ob*sity researchers find study results that undermine the "fatness is deadly" dogma of medicalized diet culture, they receive a great deal of personal and professional backlash from their peers.[4]

And, most frustrating of all, it couldn't be that all the rampant anti-fat messaging has worked so well that it has actually caused negative health outcomes for fat people. Fat people now fear shame from their doctors so much that they avoid positive health behaviors, like regular checkups. And when they do go in, doctors are encouraged by medical billing practices to treat a patient's ob*sity even if they made the appointment for tonsillitis. All of this leads to substandard medical care for fat folks. Deadly diseases like cancer are often diagnosed later in fat people, and at higher stages of development, because they were "missed" as doctors prescribed weight loss to cure initial signs and ailments.[5] And though medical fat stigma has been shown to lead to increased mortality, fat people are still blamed for their own deaths, driving the mortality statistics that serve to validate further anti-fat panic.[6]

Don't believe me? Look it up.

I did. And what I found infuriated me. Because these past forty years happen to be the ones I've been alive. So, everything that has been done to turn ob*sity from a body shape into an epidemic since 1980 has been done to my fat body. This era of fatphobia's history is incredibly personal to me.

Maybe you're stuck between those two emotions right now—anger and disbelief. Both are an opportunity.

If you are angry, sit in that anger. Let yourself stew in its juices. Baste yourself with indignation. But whatever you do, don't dismiss it. Don't you dare "yeah, but" your own internal sense that something is not right. Don't you dare stymie the power that exists in your righteous rage. Let me dispel those self-doubt demons. I offer the following two big "yeah, buts" as an exorcism, a cleansing pause before we start really digging into imagining what Fat Church could be:

"Yeah, but I don't feel good in my fat body."
Okay, do me a favor. Make a list of all the things that are difficult about living in your fat body. Everything from the difficulty of navigating dating apps to family fat jokes to the size of airline bathrooms. Write them all down. There will be a lot of items on your list, no doubt. For me there were fifty-three.

Now imagine that all structural anti-fatness has been ended in this country. Imagine that your doctors and family don't shame you anymore, that your colleagues and friends don't engage in diet talk, and that seats are sturdy everywhere you go. Imagine that clothing and employment and love and respect are all ample enough to find and to cover you. If you have a complex relationship with food, imagine it suddenly ends. Imagine trusting your body's hunger, thirst, and movement cues without filtering them through the lens of years of diet culture. Imagine being able to eat, move, and have sex for the simple pleasures these bring, without second-guessing or shame, because being fat and embodied and sexy are no longer shameful. Now reread your list as if all those structural societal changes were real. How many of your hardships remain? Likely some but far fewer.

Out of fifty-three things that I find difficult about living in my superfat body, forty-eight of them would go away if medicalized diet culture and structural anti-fatness ended tomorrow. I'm not saying life would be perfect, of course. Life isn't necessarily easy for those who live in thinner bodies. And I'd still have five hard truths about myself with which I would need to personally contend. But I do wonder if those things might be easier for me to address without the other forty-eight oppressions. Boy, would I like to know.

The point is that most fat people direct our shame and anger inward, toward our own fat as a symbol of failure, which is exactly what diet culture wants us to do. That way the industry can sell us hope in the form of another prescription, program, or procedure. When we begin to point our anger *outward*, where it belongs, at the structures of fat oppression, we can mitigate some of these things ourselves through self-advocacy and education. I have the power right now to improve twenty-two of the fifty-three items on my list, but I have to have the gumption and energy to do so. You know what fuels gumption and energy? Anger. The white-hot rage of knowing fat people deserve better. And that all people deserve freedom from anti-fatness and the body shame it causes.

"Yeah, but you're fat and so you're biased. I can't trust that anything you say is true."

Damn right I'm biased. Weight stigma limits my life and health every single day. Fat people should be listened to as experts on the experience of fatness in the same way non-white people are experts on how being racialized affects their daily lives. If you don't trust the copious amounts of research put into this book because of my dress size, that itself is a pretty solid argument that weight bias is very real, so thank you for proving my point.

I promise I didn't start my research from a place of fat acceptance, though. At the time, I was still very much mired in internalized weight stigma, worried that the medical literature would confirm all my worst fears about myself. If I'm really honest, I actually began reading medical journals as a "scared straight" tactic to try to lose weight "once and for all." So, imagine my surprise when I began finding references to "the ob*sity paradox," the medical benefits of fat, and the failure of diets to ever really work. I may have made an audible gasp.

That's why I know that this particular "yeah, but" concern is a real one. And not just from people who would, in their weight bias, deny fat people's expertise. I imagine there are people reading who desperately want to believe me and to believe that a gospel of fat liberation is good news meant for their fat bodies. But they just can't yet.

To these folks I say: I get it. A few years ago, I would have been in the exact same place.

Look to the straight-sized journalists, public health researchers, professors, and ob*sity experts who are frequently cited herein:[7] Sabrina Strings, Paul Campos, Amy Erdman Farrell, Rebecca Puhl, Traci Mann, Virginia Sole-Smith, Michelle Lelwica, Michael Hobbes, R. Marie Griffith, Lindo Bacon, and others. Look at the endnotes of this book and search for articles of interest. Begin to do the research for yourself.

Then, when you're ready to trust us fatties, start reading fat activists and cultural critics of size. Read Cat Pausé, Sonya Renee Taylor, Virgie Tovar, Hunter Ashleigh Shackelford, Sonalee Rashatwar, Caleb Luna, Da'Shaun Harrison, Aubrey Gordon, Charlotte Cooper, Rachel Wiley, Marquisele Mercedes, Joy Cox, Marilyn Wann, adrienne maree brown, Esther Rothblum, Kathleen LeBesco, Samantha Irby, Sondra Solovay, Kiese Laymon, Roxane Gay, Vanessa Rochelle Lewis, Lesley Kinzel, Jes Baker, Ilya Parker, Marianne Kirby, and Ragen Chastain,[8] just for a start. Find your story echoed in their stories, like I did. And believe them when your stories don't always align. Follow them on social media for daily doses of fat acceptance. And maybe, over time, you'll trust their voices, and maybe mine, and—most importantly—your own.

If you are stuck in disbelief, if you cannot yet believe in a gospel of fat liberation, I understand. Just please don't close yourself off from the possibility that all of this is true. Because it is. Move through your disbelief with further research. Rest in your anger and its fierce need for justice. We can be powerful agents of change. But sometimes we have to move through our disbelief in order to do so.

Moving forward to imagine Fat Church is an act of hope in something we cannot yet see: a world where fat stigma doesn't exist. "That's just a dream," you say? You're right. But so is my hope for God's reign of love and justice to be made known on the earth. So is my hope for heaven. As a Christian I choose to put my faith in things unseen all the time, as Jesus invites us to do.

CHAPTER 12:

ORIGINAL SIN, SELF-CONTROL, AND "GOOD" CHRISTIAN BODIES

Traditional Christian philosophies of the human condition are rooted in the dualist notion that one's body is a separate, lesser entity than their soul. This doctrine finds its origins in ancient Greek philosophies that predate Christianity. Early Christian theologians knew these philosophies and they filtered what they believed about Jesus through their philosophical worldviews. Many scholars see Plato's metaphysics in the writings of the Apostle Paul, for example.

Plato postulated that there's a difference between our here-and-now corporeal reality and "actual" reality, which he believed existed on another plane called the "realm of forms." According to Plato and his followers, "forms" are ideals that transcend time, inhabiting a changeless and perfect reality that exists untouched by the corruption of the material world. So, to Plato, the perfect idea of "cat" exists in the world of forms while all we can perceive here on earth are imperfect "cats," enfleshed in matter and corruptible. Earth cats merely point toward their higher ultimate form, the essential cattiest of all possible cats. No matter how sweet they are, my Simon and Jake are mere approximations, just shadows of the true ideal cat. (Please do not tell them this. They are my good, good boys.)

Plato's dualism created an ambivalence about physical bodies. They were nice and all, but they were also temporary and full of fleshy appetites and desires that must be moderated to live a good life. The soul, that eternal essence of who we are, occupies the body until the freedom of death, Plato surmised, at which time the soul is reincarnated into a different body. If a man died having lived a good life, his soul would occupy the body of another man, perhaps of higher social standing. If a man died having been a bad person, his soul would be punished by embodiment in a lesser form—a woman, or even an animal. (Which, again, really makes one wonder about cats.) Plato's dualism not only bifurcated soul and body but ranked them, with the soul being eternal and the body mortal. His notion of reincarnation of souls ranked a natural scale of living beings, with men, and men alone, at the top of the ladder.

Now think of the writings of Paul. He often talks about our present reality ending and the new reality in Christ to come. He employs those same Platonic concepts of a realm beyond our corruptible material world. In 1 Corinthians 13:12, Paul writes, "For now we see in a mirror, dimly, but then we will see face to face. Now I know only in part; then I will know fully, even as I have been fully known." Elsewhere the epistles talk of earthly concerns being "shadows of what's to come" (Colossians 2:17). Paul presents comparisons of this current, corruptible realm and its paltry concerns (like what to eat and drink, or whether to marry) with ultimate concerns like preparing for Christ's return, which Paul believed was going to happen in his lifetime. His views on women, too, were shaped by the patriarchal ordering of the world already at work in the culture of his time. Women were not quite the evolved souls that men were (echoes of Plato), and thus their bodies needed more rules to be controlled, submissive, and even silent (1 Timothy 2:11), especially owing to the "original sin"[1] of Eve.

It's important to note how Greek philosophies found their way into Paul's writings, influencing an ambiguity about mortal bodies—especially women's bodies—that would have far-reaching implications. It makes sense that Paul would be influenced by his social location. He wrote letters to bolster the individual churches he founded as a missionary in Jesus's name. All of these congregations had different populations and internal struggles. He offered masterful arguments to help these new followers get along as a countercultural community in the midst of an empire. Later, imitators used the clout of Paul's name to write additional letters, which spread alongside his original words as explanations of how to live a righteous life. Christian theology was moving from situational instructions for waiting out the soon-expected return of Christ[2] to a "Christian way of life" morality.

Future theologians interpreted Paul's words and the life of Jesus from their own cultural standpoints. They utilized the same dualistic philosophy, often describing the spiritual struggle to free the soul from the grips of the sinful body.[3] Many Early Church Fathers[4] pointed especially to women's bodies as the source of corporeal corruption. Like Paul, they traced the lineage of sin all the way back to the Garden of Eden, to the first woman, Eve.

Original Sin and Women's Bodies

The first sin recorded in our scriptures is a woman disobeying authority by putting a forbidden food to her lips and taking a big bite. And the first consequence of that sin is body shame.

In Genesis 3:1–24, we see Eve tricked by the serpent into eating the fruit of the "Tree of the Knowledge of Good and Evil," the one tree in all of the Garden of Eden from which God says not to eat. She then shares that fruit with Adam, who also eats. They immediately recognize that they are naked, sew up some quick fig leaf couture, and, in their shame, hide from God.

God's first question to them is "who told you that you were naked?" an indication that body shame was never meant to be part of God's good Creation. For their mistake, Adam and Eve are forever spoiled from their eternal paradise and thrust into mortal life. Adam will have to use his body to toil the earth to eat and survive. Eve will endure the pain of childbirth and—bonus penance—be afraid of snakes.

As part of their expulsion, God expressly makes Adam "ruler" over his woman. This harkens back to the second Creation narrative in Genesis 2:4–25, where God forms woman from Adam's rib after noticing Adam's need for companionship. In this second account of Creation, woman is not formed as her own being but as a complimentary "help-mate" for Adam, an extension of his own body. Thus, God's admonition in Genesis 3:16 for Adam to "rule" over his wife serves to reinforce the "complementarian"[5] Creation narrative in which Eve is not a subject on her own, but an object under the headship of Adam. Adam is even the one who gives Eve her name, not God.

With dualism (the hierarchy of soul over body) on the one hand and complementarianism (women are not subjects but objects) on the other, female bodies became sites of great consternation and church control. Feminist theologians Lisa Isherwood and Elizabeth Stewart offer this description of the consequences of the second story of Creation, determining it not only to be the source of how women are understood in society, but how they understand themselves:

> [I]t is a myth that has set the theological agenda for women and our bodies. An agenda that is still impacting on us today. The rib, once removed, becomes an object, an "other," quite separate from God's original creation, man. This is to be the role of woman in religion and theology, to act as the "other," the outsider, to the holy trinity of man, God and church. Man is the norm of creation and woman never quite measures up; all that is unique about her is seen as somehow defective and suspect. She is taught to mistrust herself, particularly the knowledge that she gains through her "guts," her body knowing.[6]

Here's where some Early Church Fathers loved to riff, concerning themselves deeply with the problem of women. To them, Eve gave women their dangerous physicality.[7] She is the first temptress but far from the last. Tertullian's first-century *De Cultu Feminarium* instructs Christian women to dress modestly to visually connote their repentance for the sin of Eve, which, passed down through time, now resides within them. He argues:

> Do you not know that you are (each) an Eve? The sentence of God on this sex of yours lives in this age: the guilt must of necessity live too. *You* are the devil's gateway: *you* are the unsealer of that (forbidden) tree: *you* are the first deserter of the divine law: *you* are she who persuaded him whom the devil was not valiant enough to attack. *You* destroyed so easily God's image, man. On account of *your* desert—that is, death—even the Son of God had to die. And do you think about adorning yourself over and above your tunics of skins? Come, now.[8]

Christian theology and history, mostly developed and passed down by men, became filled with expositions on the corruption Eve let loose on the world and, thus, the need for women to be controlled. Saint Jerome's writings, for example, are fun to read with a nice white wine in a bubble bath—pair *Adversus Jovinian* with a buttery pinot grigio. Therein Jerome couches his expositions on virginity and marriage within the narrative of the Fall and philosophy of dualism. Women show their "inner man" when they can remain chaste, putting things of the spirit and mind above the lusts of the body, and even in marriage the touch of one's wife is potentially corrupting to a man's soul.[9]

Religious asceticism grew in popularity, especially in monastic communities where women could be avoided altogether. For a righteous Christian life, sexual lust was, of course, a big no-no, but so were things like taking too much pleasure in one's food, having hot baths, or even smelling too nice; any opportunity for the senses to run amok invited earthly temptations that could put one's soul in danger.[10] Saint Augustine, writing to a Christian man who had decided to leave a monastery at his mother's behest, offers, "Watch out that [your mother] does not twist and overturn you for the worse. What difference does it make whether it is in a wife or in a mother, provided that we nonetheless avoid Eve in any woman?"[11] To Augustine, the earthly, carnal love of a woman could be tempting even if maternal in nature.

Founders within the early church mistrusted the female body and formulated theological writings, religious rules, and wider society to make her perform her power only for men's sake (procreation) and under their watchful gaze (marriage). Even a woman's voice could lead men astray, as was the case with Adam. The fourth-century Archbishop of Constantinople, John Chrysostom, reinforced Paul's admonition in 1 Timothy for women to remain silent, saying:

> The [female] sex is naturally somewhat talkative: and for this reason [Paul] restrains them on all sides. "For Adam," says [Paul], "was first formed, then Eve. And Adam was not deceived, but the woman being deceived was in the transgression." If it be asked, what has this to do with women of the present day? It shows that the male sex enjoyed the higher honor. Man was first formed; and elsewhere [Paul] shows their superiority. "Neither was the man created for the woman, but the woman for the man." (1 Corinthians 11:9) Why then does [Paul] say this? He wishes the man to have the preeminence in every way . . . For the woman [Eve] taught the man once, and made him guilty of disobedience, and wrought our ruin. Therefore, because she made a bad use of her power over

the man, or rather her equality with him, God made her subject to her husband.[12]

As lusty, earthly bodies, women were by their nature able to continue the species, and it was Eve's self-willed agency that led to humanity's corruption in the first place.[13] For this reason, the "Eve" within every woman must remain under male control. Michelle Lelwica explains these patriarchal fears, saying:

> For centuries, male Christian leaders argued that the damning consequences of Eve's agency "proved" women were not suited for leadership but should be confined to the domestic sphere, where they could pursue a career of consecrated virginity, or fulfill their divinely sanctioned duty of procreating children and serving their husbands. The slippage between Eve and the generic "woman" in these writings implied that all women are blameworthy, untrustworthy, and deserving of shame . . . Though men's bodies were also seen as suspect among the church fathers, the most serious contempt was reserved for unruly female flesh.[14]

These efforts to control women's bodily behaviors are the roots of "purity culture," still very much alive and well today. We can hear early church echoes of female disobedience any time a victim of sexual assault is asked what she was wearing, or when a woman who claims her own sexuality is deemed a "slut." Some Christian fathers still today give their preteen daughters "purity rings," a physical symbol of male ownership over female sexuality.

This same objectification and control of women also allows men to be the judges of women's performance of femininity, instead of women determining for themselves what femininity means to them. The laundry list of aesthetic, spiritual, and physical practices that women "are supposed to" perform is known by its shorthand, "beauty." Naomi Wolf's *The Beauty Myth* describes it thusly:

> Genesis explains why it is women who often need to offer their bodies to any male gaze that will legitimize them. "Beauty" now gives the female body the legitimacy that God withheld . . . Women tend to worry about physical perfection in a way men seldom do because Genesis says that all men are created perfect, whereas Woman began as an inanimate piece of meat; malleable, unsculpted, unauthorized, raw—imperfect.[15]

Here Augustine might very well agree with Wolf's assessment, given his reflection:

> The woman together with her own husband is the image of God, so that that whole substance may be one image; but when she is referred separately to her quality of help-meet, which regards the woman herself alone, then she is not the image of God; but as regards the man alone, he is the image of God as fully and completely as when the woman too is joined with him in one.[16]

But women were not wholly doomed. By medieval times, the church began to acknowledge female saints, often cloistered women acting in penance for Eve's original sin by practicing chastity, meekness, and mortification of flesh.[17] These women took responsibility for their own spiritual discipline, a means of agency despite the rules of patriarchal culture. Anorexia, in particular, was considered a saintly gesture for women, their fasting evidence of an ability to deny earthly hungers in favor of spiritual gains.[18]

The thinner the woman, the closer to God she supposedly became through her ability to put "mind over matter," a dualistic cliché still in use that Saint Jerome would have loved. Fat bodies, on the other hand, were considered examples of gluttonous appetites fulfilled.[19] Body size became a visual cue for moral goodness or badness, virtue or sin.

Michelle Lelwica also notes the effects of eschatology, or theologies about God's judgment at the "end times" and of heaven, in the historical notion of the "good" Christian body.[20] Lelwica outlines how earthly bodies, with their mortality and corruption, were imagined to become eternal, spiritual bodies in the afterlife— perfect bodies no longer encumbered by illness, pain, or death.[21] This became part of the very nature of Christian "salvation." By believing in Christ and becoming baptized as one with the Body of Christ on earth—the church—humans could anticipate that day beyond today when all their earthly corruption would be redeemed. Lelwica says:

> By equating bodily redemption with physical perfection, early church leaders systemically removed somatic impairments, afflictions, and irregularities from God's kingdom. In so doing, they implicitly conflated disease, deformity, and disability with sin, impurity, and punishment. Ultimately, this eschatological cleansing interpreted bodily anomalies and ailments as signs of corruption in God's perfect creation . . . This eschatological nostalgia for wholeness echoes in the longing to "get back to normal" described by some people living with chronic illness or pain, disability, or the process of aging. Whether the ideal body that orients this thinking is located in the past (e.g. "before I got sick") or future (e.g. "when I'm cured"), the mentality itself diverts our attention away

from the present and makes it very difficult to feel at peace in a body that refuses to be cured or improved.[22]

And, of course, the life of Jesus and his miraculous healings, in their traditional reading,[23] seemed to give credence to this understanding of history.[24] According to the gospels, Jesus enabled the blind to see and the disabled to walk. His miracles became a central feature of his earthly ministry and were understood to be a foretaste of God's reordering of earth to come, all things made new. This is an eschatological promise, the promise of a heaven without illness. Understood in the light of "perfect" heavenly bodies to come, Jesus's cures were not just of people's ailments but also their mortal souls. "Your faith has made you well,"[25] and "go and sin no more"[26] are utterances from Jesus's lips that seem to equate bodily ills with spiritual ones.[27]

It's not difficult to imagine the devastating effects this theology had on the treatment of anyone whose bodies strayed from what was considered "normal" (read: "good") as defined by the church.[28] Any malady could be assumed to be the result of God's judgment for some wanton sin. Priests and other arbiters of God were required to have bodies within the norms of society or could not serve.[29] The church's teachings suggested that "a body's external contours, abilities, and features manifest a person's internal moral character."[30]

Conversely, some theologians lifted up illness and disability as "redemptive suffering," still moralized but this time as a test from God. Understood thusly, the chronically ill and disabled could be seen paternalistically as spiritually *exceptional* for the ways their very existence was a permanent mortification of the flesh they must "endure" for the one-day promise of a perfect body in heaven.[31] Christian "charity" toward those with both physical and mental disabilities historically took the form of institutionalization, keeping disabled folks away from society altogether. While this sequestration provided some families an escape from suspicions of sin and societal judgment, it often meant a difficult life of neglect and abuse for the disabled person.[32]

Both disability theologians and secular crip theorists[33] reject these notions of moral "goodness" or "sinfulness" and emphasize the disabled person as their own agent in the world, rather than an objective symbol of righteousness or damnation for others' judgment.[34] It should be noted that fat studies and disability studies align in this way, since both sets of bodies are seen as culturally abject and often need accommodations to fully inhabit society.[35]

We modern Christians may be tempted to imagine that we have moved beyond the harmful body philosophies of the early church. We may scoff at the fact that, in medieval times, a woman who birthed a child with health issues was interrogated about her sins, or the midwife's transgressions were blamed.[36] Either way, female sinfulness was at fault. But Louise Gosbell warns that this thinking is still very much alive today. She points to the enormous cultural expectations on women to perform a healthy pregnancy by all manner of rituals: taking folic acid, not smoking, eating or not eating certain foods, not being too old or unfit, and undergoing batteries of medical tests to determine the child's genetics and healthy development.[37] Though these measures of motherly virtue now operate under the watchful eye of a secular doctor rather than the clergy, their performance is sacrosanct and the punchline is the same: a woman is often considered "to blame" for any health problems that arise.

Louise Gosbell asks:

> How much do statements such as, "It doesn't matter if it is a boy or a girl,[38] as long as it's healthy" from those within faith communities reveal the pervasiveness of the belief

that human value is something to be achieved through physical and intellectual potential rather than something that is imbued?[39]

Theologians of disability would here join Gosbell's critique, since what she calls the "idolatry of normality"[40] is pervasive in American culture.

There is intrinsic sacred value in all bodies. It is also true that Christians believe something lies beyond these mortal desires of ours, a broader narrative that moves us past ourselves into communion with the Divine. So, throughout the Christian story, many theologians and everyday saints have emphasized a denial of our bodily hungers. Only when we deny ourselves, they've said, can true spiritual understanding arise.

But what if our mortal desires are not sinful things from which we must be freed, but signposts toward even greater communion and revelation? What if God wants our bodies, in all their copiousness and want, to be fully satisfied? What if this generosity is part of God's good gifts to all of Creation? What if soul and body are inextricably connected?

A new Christian spirituality emerges within the work of fat liberation. It invites us to embrace the values of abundance, goodness, and structural justice for all bodies as alternatives to the values of scarcity, sinfulness, and individual responsibility that underlie diet culture and anti-fatness. This spirituality revels in bodily pleasure, emotion, beauty, and even lust—things too often denigrated by the church as wildly feminine and animalistic. But we all feel their pull. To some, this universality of experience points to the truth of the doctrine of Original Sin. In a spirituality of fat liberation, though, the invitation to enjoy the fullness of our bodies, to revel in our flesh, is part and parcel of what it means to experience a full life in God's good Creation.

This is no wanton pipe dream. It's a faithful reading of scripture, albeit one wrested away from traditional Christian interpretations of the human body. The values of abundance, goodness, and structural justice for all bodies are just as central to the Christian narrative as the themes from which anti-fatness emerged. And the life and ministry of Jesus is an invitation to reorder society away from a cultural hierarchy of bodies, toward liberative relationships with our own and others' bodies, rooted in God's abundance for all.

THE PARABLE OF THE WEEDS

I read a poem once that spoke of the change of heart and mind that must come before true acceptance.[1] The author looks at the weedy mess of her home garden, its unruliness. She knows the backbreaking work she must do to get her garden back to "good order." She must go to her knees in the dirt, pulling every offensive weed out by the root lest it grow back in the same place again. She must sweat and toil and exert her control over the garden to make it finally beautiful.

The poet doesn't want to do this work. She wants to enjoy her day and, upon inspection, the weeds aren't actually as ugly as they're made out to be. They're pretty, in fact. Fairly miraculous, too, in the way they fight for their right to be there, their right to take up space in the garden even when unwanted.

So, she looks in the dictionary and finds that the definition of a weed is "any unwelcome plant." Flinging her home's back door open wide, she stands on her porch and yells out toward the garden, "You are all welcome here!"

Then, miraculously, she has no more weeds. This is an act of revolutionary hospitality.

Taking on a gospel of body liberation necessitates such a world-changing reframing.

CHAPTER 13:

JESUS AND THE RELUCTANT SAINTS OF FAT LIBERATION

I have read lots of memoirs and manifestos from righteous fat babes. It seems they always include their corporeal pedigree, snapshots of navigating their body's homegoing to itself and/or how they left societal shame behind. I love reading these stories because they are often so recognizable. With commiseration I laugh at weight-loss plans gone wrong, and I cry at descriptions of being bullied as "less than" because of being so much more. Both are familiar to me. It's no wonder that fat activism has rooted itself in storytelling.[1]

Since the beginning of the fat rights movement in the late 1960s, fat activists have produced an enormous number of publications telling their own stories of living large. Many of these were never meant to go mainstream, having been personal letters or self-published zines in the early days. For this reason, most are truly countercultural. They're unfiltered and deliciously filthy in their disregard for respectability. They were aimed at their target audiences, people often marginalized by American society not only for their fatness but because of their sexuality, gender expression, social class, perceived race, employment, ethnicity, and/or ability. From its beginning, fat activism has thus understood itself to be an intersectional movement, which has made personal stories all the more important sources of understanding.

In the 1990s, the internet began providing space for blogs, websites, and chatrooms where fat people gathered in community. These began to bring the work of fat activism, and the voices of fat people, further into society. This much-ridiculed effort toward fat pride has drawn ire from journalists, doctors, the diet industry, as well as everyday Americans struggling to understand fat people as anything more than failed thin people.[2] Still, the brave work of self-advocacy among early fat activists, their refusal to shrink or comply with diet culture, has paved the way for fat to be increasingly understood as a valid marker of identity. Their stories surface what it means to be fat in society and dignify fat self-acceptance, both of which greatly improve the lives of fat people and others marginalized by their bodies' noncompliance with white hegemonic beauty and wellness culture.[3]

Fat narratives undermine the tropes of fatness so prevalent in our everyday lives. The accounts of how hard people have worked to lose weight and yet failed not only cast doubt on the efficacy of diets themselves but on the notion of the lazy fat person with no willpower. A raunchy narrative of fat sexuality contrasts with society's notion that no one finds fat bodies desirable. Memoirs of cooking and eating unashamedly for pleasure and comfort remind us all that food is not just a mechanistic way to nourish our body-machines but a universal goodness shared by all people and all cultures. Fat stories told by fat people are an important means of cultural disruption and a call to a more abundant life.

Imagining Fat Church

The concept of *Fat Church* first arose as I explored these early writings of fat activists. They were so brave and unabashed in their countercultural messages. Their movement started in embodied practices and surreptitious gatherings outside of the mainstream. Their words spread in personal correspondence and oral histories that were then saved and reproduced, a growing wave of thought emerging from the margins. Some collected these thoughts, seeing the complexity and the contradictions within them not as faults but as natural tessellations of truth that bore witness to the emergence of repeated patterns. Further authors built upon these archived writings. They created a field of inquiry interested in uncovering ways to better society with greater understanding, greater inclusion, and greater compassion for self and others.

To my pastoral ears, this sounded a whole lot like the early church. I know; I know. Leave it to a Christian clergyperson to see Jesus everywhere. But, by God, I did see him.

Jesus cared that people were fed and fed well. His miracles often focused on food. At his mother's behest, Jesus's first miracle yielded the finest wine to save a wedding's hospitality. His most attested miracle fed multitudes of people from miraculous abundance—a few fish and loaves of bread feeding 5,000 people, with baskets of leftovers. This particular story is told six different times in the span of four gospels, meaning two of the books contain the narrative twice. Such is its importance. Jesus communed with those his society considered unclean and undesirable in defiance of custom, but in the promise of a more inclusive day to come. When he knew his death was near, Jesus left his followers an embodied form of remembrance in a simple meal of bread and wine. In these ways, eating became for Jesus a sign of the Reign of God to come, the inbreaking of another era. Abundant life. And when Jesus returned from death, he showed himself to his disciples by cooking breakfast, and by breaking bread in their midst once again. They recognized him through his hospitality.

This is why I saw Jesus in fat activists' invitation to eat joyfully, without shame, and to the point of satisfaction. I saw him in their community gatherings where all were welcome and ample space was made for bodily accommodations. I heard Jesus's teachings echoed as fat people named themselves beloved when society named them otherwise. I saw his righteous anger in fat activist resistance and protests, the bold smallness of their collective voice a perpetual underdog against the empire of monied diet culture. But mostly I saw Jesus weeping with the stories of fat people's pain.

I imagined him angry at the vitriol of anti-fat hatred and violence done to bodies in the name of "health." I saw Jesus beckoning society toward a different way. He was beckoning me toward a different relationship with my own fat body. I even dared to imagine Jesus himself fat, filling out every bit of his 5XL robes. Majestic.

Despite these visions of mine, fat activism certainly hasn't been a Christian endeavor to date. It wasn't founded as a religious movement at all, and doubtless many fat activists would take exception to my seeing Jesus in their work. In fact, fat activists specifically name the Christian church as an institution unyielding in its denigration of bodily appetites of all sorts, which makes it a happy bedfellow with diet culture (albeit a chaste bedfellow, of *course*). Fat activists describe suffering some of their most wounding anti-fat critiques within the churches of their youth. These critiques rang true to me, having experienced a maddening many myself.

I grew up in the Bible Belt. Like most belts, it never seemed to fit me just right. Where I'm from you ask what church someone attends early in the conversation as a means of understanding both who they are and who they know. Church is a socio-spiritual enterprise in many locales, but on the well-manicured streets of suburban West Tennessee, your congregational identity marks you with genus-and-species specificity. So, when I say I was a white, middle-class United Methodist, you should realize this meant my personal piety was somewhere between Southern Baptist and Episcopalian. As the old joke goes, this meant fellow congregants would say hello to you in the liquor store, but only if you were both buying a nice wine. We always dressed up for church, sat in the same pew each week, and hoped the preacher didn't go overboard on the sermon. We didn't want the Presbyterians beating us to the Cracker Barrel.

Church was our entire social circle. We attended Sunday morning worship, Sunday night youth group, Wednesday night Bible study and choir practice, with occasional events speckled across other days of the week. White, Southern Protestant Christianity flavored my worldview. Every belief I had about myself and others was filtered through its lens. This shaped my understanding of what it meant to be a good person. To be acceptable in the eyes of my church was to be acceptable in the eyes of God.

I cannot count the number of times the "your body is a temple" scripture from 1 Corinthians 6:19–20 was proof-texted to me as either an admonition of my failure to become thin or as an invitation to try again. No joke, when I Googled "Bible your body is a temple" to find the verse number, the very first result that came up was an article from my hometown newspaper.[4] I had to laugh out loud. And it's ripe with all the churchy body shaming I remember: a cutesy joke about the "battle of the bulge," an admonition against "not participating in that which is of the carnal nature," and an underlying dualism that pits flesh against spirit. Some things never change.

In my youth, I had sweet Christian matriarchs of my church pinch my growing sides, offering me the dire prophesy that I'd never find a husband at my size. Marriage, to them, was the primary goal of womanhood. (And when I did get married, their worry immediately shifted to my fertility.) I navigated every coffee hour, potluck, and funeral collation under the watchful eye of those who saw my body as the consequence of cardinal sins—gluttony and sloth—and I grabbed an extra brownie accordingly, in chocolatey defiance.[5] Pastors took me aside to warn me specifically about another cardinal sin, lust, since my body was developing earlier and more amply than my peers. I needed to dress even more modestly, even more carefully than thinner girls whose bodies had not yet filled out. I heard corpses body shamed at their own funerals, "It was her weight that did her in. Bless her heart." I joined church-sponsored dieting and exercise groups where women became one another's accountability partners to make sure none of us strayed from our righteous regimens. When someone "backslid" I heard them utter tearful cupcake confessions, asking Jesus for forgiveness from their sin. All of this was earnest. None of it was helpful.

This was in the church of my younger days. One might be tempted to think with my move from the South to the Northeast, into a more progressive Christian denomination, experiences of anti-fat bias would have subsided. In some ways, yes. The combination of growing much fatter and becoming clergy means no one in my church has critiqued my size to my face for some time. For that I am exceedingly grateful. But I still hear the disparaging comments that people make about their own *much smaller* weights.[6] I pass the "Overeaters Anonymous" meeting that happens in our church weekly and see women sitting in the same circle formation I remember from my youth, sharing their struggles to become or stay thin. I hear people moralize their food choices, saying things like, "I was good at lunch so I'm going to have just a little slice of cake." If I use the word "fat" to describe myself, people offer the old chestnut, "You're not fat! You're beautiful," revealing an inherently anti-fat sentiment.[7] I see clergy health initiatives published by my and other Christian denominations that equate thinness with health and weight loss with self-care. I notice a local clergy group has committed to attending Weight Watchers together and they post their weekly accountability on Facebook for all to see. I do not care that Rev. So-and-so backslid with an apple fritter. Yet collectively they get hundreds of positive comments on their "progress." I hear from a distraught fat colleague that he was asked in his ordination boards, within a liberal denomination, "How can you be a good role model for your church at that size?"

The people inhabiting both my childhood and current churches are beloved, faithful, good folks. Most would never want to hurt me nor anyone else for that matter. Casual anti-fatness slips by unnoticed, everyone unaware of how small messages—little things that seem so fleeting—have lasting consequences and serve to bolster cultural weight stigma and body shame. And they especially don't think of the children overhearing them talk, taking in every comment like I did to build a woefully sizeist Christian worldview.

And, sadly, these people are not being un-Christian, not at all. We've recounted how anti-fat bias arose alongside Christian teachings on the body's failings and lusts (especially among women), and how the soul's salvation was imagined to be found in the heaven of perfect health. We've seen how the elite, white Protestants (WASPs) who "settled" America brought with them a Christian patriarchal culture rooted in understanding all bodily appetites as downright dangerous to society, especially when embodied by the non-WASP immigrant groups growing around them. Thus, moderation came to be understood as the key to being both "healthy" and a "good, civilized Christian."

Together, these distillations of historic Christian teachings (anti-woman, anti-body, pro-moderation) became the foundation blocks of modern-day American anti-fatness. And this truth always has been directed most pointedly toward the fat female form, she who has been the church's favorite scapegoat since Eve first bit that apple.

CHAPTER 14:

JESUS HEALS A WOMAN

Let me re-tell you a story.

She hadn't been in a crowd this size for a long, long time. Twelve years, in fact. She was grateful for the way its crush made her inconspicuous, a luxury she didn't usually enjoy. The offense of her body was an embarrassment that demanded isolation and control. Deemed unclean, she was a contagious threat to her society. But on this day, she moved through the multitude, misbehaving out of necessity, even as she anticipated the commotion she could cause if spotted.

Luckily, all eyes were on him. Some had come out of curiosity and others out of desperation. All of them wondered about this strange rabbi who healed as he taught, promising a new world to come. That's what she was looking for, a new world in which her unruly body could be different. A chance at a life lived as fully as possible.

She had tried everything she could on her own. Doctors repeatedly promised her recovery with just another treatment, just another intervention. Their promises were as bankrupt as she now was from their care. Nothing she did worked. Maybe her transgression today, here in the crowd, would. She touched everyone around her, elbows and hips taking up every inch of room she could to get to him. She reached out her hand, straining against the other bodies to touch his robe as he walked past. It was worth a shot.

Fat liberation is about healing, something about which we Christians are supposed to know. Our scriptures are full of instances of miraculous healings. Traditionally understood, these are stories of bodies "made whole" by their encounters with Jesus. The Acts of the Apostles, those earliest accounts of the Christian movement, are made wondrous by their descriptions of yet more interventions on behalf of bodies. Enacted by the power of the Spirit, these are meant to be a foretaste of what's to come in the heaven of someday.

The story of Jesus healing a bleeding woman is told three different times in the Christian gospels: Mark 5:25–34, Matthew 9:20–22, and Luke 8:43–48.

Here's Mark's version of the story:

> Now there was a woman who had been suffering from hemorrhages for twelve years. She had endured much under many physicians, and had spent all that she had; and she was no better, but rather grew worse. She had heard about Jesus, and came up behind him in the crowd and touched his cloak, for she said, "If I but touch his clothes, I will be made well." Immediately her hemorrhage stopped; and she felt in her body that she was healed of her disease. Immediately aware that power had gone forth from him, Jesus turned about in the crowd and said, "Who touched my clothes?" And his disciples said to him, "You see the crowd pressing in on you; how can you say, 'Who touched me?'" He looked all around to see who had done it. But the woman, knowing what had happened to her, came in fear and trembling, fell down before him, and told him the whole truth. He said to her, "Daughter, your faith has made you well; go in peace, and be healed of your disease."
> – Mark 5:25–34

Though she is nameless, her story is familiar. A woman fed up, desperate. A woman ready to try something—anything—new to finally control her uncontrollable body. She has arbitrated herself in every which way, consulting doctors, religious authorities, and the homemade wisdoms that women pass down in secret to one another from generation to generation. Still the blood came; for twelve years it came. She didn't know there could be so much within her. She would have happily laid it as a blood sacrifice on any altar that would make her well. She had given everything up for the sake of her own repair, spared no expense, endured whatever the doctors threw at her. Still, nothing but blood and shame and isolation from her society, which considered bodies like hers unclean.

I can't help but imagine her to be a big, fat woman. A woman like me.

In her story I hear echoes of my own nonstop attempts to "heal" from the problem of my body. Told by doctors, family, and society for years that my copious weight is a deadly hindrance, I have laid money, time, blood, sweat, and tears at the altar of diet culture, begging for something to break me open and rescue the thin woman promised to be inside of me. I have been told always to heal myself, to shrink into submission. In this effort I have failed repeatedly. For a dozen years, or twenty, I got used to the shame of knowing this was my own fault, and trying yet again. Dismayed by the permanence of our fat bodies, fat folks do as the bleeding woman did, trying prescribed remedies over and over again to "heal," yet never finding absolution.

I try to imagine a woman of 350 pounds being hemmed in by the crowd that day, looking for Jesus. She is used to her body being compressed by girdles, the arms of chairs, clothing that doesn't come in her size, but she isn't used to such an assembly pressing in on her. Strangers usually avoid her touch. She stood on the bus to get here because all the seats were taken by purses and bags, the stares of passengers communicating their dread of her big body as their seatmate. She had to take the bus, since planes charge people her size for two seats. She is used to being bumped into, jostled by strangers who misjudge her girth and walk away without apology. She is always at fault for the bigness of her body.

Here, in this crowd, she does not shrink herself. She does not hang at the back edge of the photo to hide her magnitude behind others, but instead pushes her way forward. For once, her size is an asset, and she makes it to the front of the line. Still, stretching out her arm, she hopes not to be noticed. She hates being noticed. But she does want healing. So, she touches him. Not him, really. She doesn't want to be a bother. Just his robe. Just the hem, even. With hope she thinks maybe this time it'll be different.

The big question is what, then, does Jesus do? Feeling his power leave him, turning to her, what does he see? What does "healing" even mean for her fat body? Does it mean thinness, a sudden miraculous deflation? The kind we are all looking for in our thirty-day cleanses and clean eating regimens? Jesus, the ultimate dietician? If she suddenly loses the weight, does it stay off forever, or does she have to have the willpower "not to sin again"?

> He looked all around to see who had done it. But the woman, knowing what had happened to her, came in fear and trembling, fell down before him, and told him the whole truth. He said to her, "Daughter, your faith has made you well; go in peace, and be healed of your disease."
> – Mark 5:32–34

I imagine this fat woman falling to her knees, pouring her heart out to Jesus. I see the crowd murmuring its disapproval. She should get out of the way, that woman who clearly did this to herself. She should step aside and let those *actual* disabled people[1] behind her reach Jesus. The audacity of asking for a sudden healing! What laziness! How dare she ask Jesus for something that could so easily be hers for the reasonable price of a gym membership in perpetuity and a little willpower! Someone snaps a cell phone photo of her on the ground, groveling. He posts it with the tags #cow, #moo, #lol, and, ironically, #bodypositivity, just to make sure other fat folks see it and know their place.

I am this woman, of course. Maybe you are too. Anyone, fat or thin, who has been shamed for a body outside of the "norms" of their culture feels this struggle to be changed. To fit in.

Except I don't think that Jesus healed bodies so they could assimilate into the society that once shunned them. What good is blending into the *status quo*? What a small goal that would have been. In that light, Jesus's healings would have helped a few people feel better. It would have helped them regain access to some of what they had lost as outcasts. But according to the scriptures he only healed a few. What of the others left wanting?

No, Jesus came for the cause of liberation, not assimilation. His message of inclusion wasn't into the established hierarchies of empire but into God's infinite hospitality. *There is room for you. There is room for all of Creation.* God's embodied inbreaking is pointed toward another society altogether, whose new principles we saw enacted in the radical life of Jesus: hospitable abundance and generosity, communal care and friendship, pleasure and appreciation, self-sacrifice and, yes, healing. Healing not for those unfortunate, "othered" bodies, but for us all.

Collective Healing

The healing stories that pepper our scriptures have been used by the Christian church throughout its history to objectify, belittle, and abuse people whose bodies fall outside of the "norm."[2] Since the fourth century, Christianity has been an authoritative voice in defining culture, often dictating its ingroups and outgroups. These striations have served to prop up empire rather than undermine it.

Still worse, the church has theologized itself into harrowing abuses of people whose bodies were thought of as "less-than" because of their differences. In the US, for example, this has taken form in the sin of white supremacy, our Protestant settlers happily embracing the eradication of Indigenous peoples and the enslavement of Africans to make their one nation, under God, prosperous.

Jesus did not come to heal people toward participation in such an existing state of affairs but to free us from it. But what might a new society look like? And how might we get there?

Theologian Shelly Rambo speaks of deep societal wounds such as the festering effects of racism in America.[3] Offering a glimpse of what might support shared healing, Rambo suggests, "a wound remains, untended, below the surface of the collective skin. Coming to terms with history involves a spiritual reckoning and a process of unraveling the stories that were told about why things are the way they are."[4] Such a "spiritual reckoning" must include bearing witness to the wounds, naming or hearing the violence of them, and facing their depths.[5] We know this to be true about bodies. If a wound is not fully healed from within, patching its surface will not end the decay.

An effort could be made to surface the church's participation in structural racism, which might in turn support societal healing. But instead, most expressions of American Christianity offer what Rambo calls a "sacred bandage,"[6] a gauze meant to both placate and obscure realities the church never actually intends to heal. She says, "Christianity claims to offer healing, but in fact it is implicated in covering up and covering over wounds that lie below the surface. If and when they are surfaced, Christianity does not allow them to be exposed to the light."[7] It is a fragile faith that cannot excavate wounds of its own making. But this is exactly what happens, for example, when some Christians hide behind bland scriptural statements of "in Christ we are all one body" while denying that structural racism exists.

The church must wrestle with the ways its ideologies have often propagated societal ills. Rambo's "spiritual reckoning" offers an alternative vision to ignoring, and thus further marginalizing, those whose wounds must be acknowledged for any chance at societal healing. It hurts to do this work. It is messy and ongoing, likely never fully complete. What even is "healing" then in the context of deep societal wounds such as racism and its counterpart, sizeism?[8]

To Rambo, healing is not a one-time, individual, triumphant physical overcoming; it's a lasting communal effort, guided by the Spirit, which invites fearless encounters with wounds and truth-telling about how they arose in the first place.[9] Such was Jesus's intention, Rambo posits, when he offered his own post-resurrection wounds so boldly to Thomas and the disciples in the Upper Room.[10] *Do not be afraid. Touch my wounds. Stop doubting and believe.*[11] It is a communal invitation to healing, not just an individual one.

The woman is still there, on the ground, by the way. She is kneeling at Jesus's side, awaiting a word from him. The crowd's chatter dies down and he speaks: "Daughter, your faith has made you well; go in peace, and be healed of your disease."[12]

In this important moment, I do not believe that her fat body shrinks. I believe her shame does. *Because the disease was the shame all along.*

She has poured her story out to Jesus, the only one in the crowd who sees her as fully as she sees herself. He has listened unflinchingly to her truth. To him, this fat woman is a "subject" in her own right, rather than an outcast "object" on which others write their stereotypes or society's fears.

She has "told him the whole truth" (v.33), something fat people are not encouraged to do. We are the chubby sidekick to the main character with a few funny lines but never a true narrative. We are either the bridesmaid or the other woman. We are told to keep our mouths shut, that we should be grateful for the attention. We are often assumed to have no voice at all, no heads even, just torsos of epidemic proportions.[13] Our stories are told for us, usually through the lens of our weight-loss struggles, the hardships we face fitting into a society made for the small. Our fat guts are opened wide for the camera, a spectacle of flesh. But we are to keep our mouths shut.

Fat people are thought to be capital-T tragic. But this is not the truth of our lives, no matter how many seasons and spinoffs of *My 600-lb Life* there are. We cannot be reduced.

Fat people, like all "othered" people, live complex lives worthy of dignity and care. Cultural anti-fat bias tries to remove that dignity and care by replacing it with shame and dismissal. A Rambo-esque "spiritual reckoning" is necessary to open up the wound of anti-fat hate in our society and see what lies beneath, as she says, by "unraveling the stories that were told about why things are the way they are."[14]

Much of this truth-telling takes us into medical and public health spaces that we don't typically dare to go as fat people. We have done this work in this manuscript, and the punchline is that fat bodies are not abject failures of willpower, destined for an early grave. Those misconceptions do tremendous damage to our psyches and wellbeing.

We have also peeled back the sacred bandage over white Anglo-Saxon Protestantism and gazed at the ways it has ordered American society toward both racism and anti-fat bias, two ills inextricably linked in our culture.[15] We have unraveled a few of the theological stories long told by the church that blame women for bodily corruption, rendering all her appetites suspect.

We must all be brave and gentle with ourselves and others as we do this work. (We do not have to be gentle with the culture, though. That's where our collective anger, power, and activism belongs.) Thinner people and small-fats must not flinch as they face wounds they have never experienced themselves, things that may seem difficult to believe if it weren't for such widespread evidence. Larger fats like me must be brave enough to confront the reality that sustained weight loss is not likely and *fatness is a valid and permanent identity*. This can be terrifying when all one has ever wanted is to be "normal," to be "healed," to be "acceptable." These are traps. They are not enough.

I invite you to want *more* than this. You deserve more than to be assimilated into the society that didn't want you fifty pounds ago, and that will drop you the second you gain it all back.

Fat people, it's time to live unashamed and whole, just as we are. Let us reach out past assimilation, past even body positivity, to touch true body liberation's hem.

THE PANTRY

There was a kitchen in the household of my youth. And within that kitchen there was a pantry. And in that pantry, there were shelves. And on those shelves lay all manner of provisions, every one of which was an approved food of whatever latest diet my family was enduring.

For two years our pantry was filled with "foods" from Nutrisystem, and let me tell you there is nothing that makes you stare into the existential void more quickly than shelf-stable dehydrated beef patties. I spent the tenderloin of my youth, ages twelve to fourteen, bringing to school lunches so strange and harrowing that even I didn't want to sit with me. I would say it was space food but there are no fat astronauts. No, it was food from a dystopian future ruled by thin overlords[*] hellbent on punishing fat people by removing all sense of taste, texture, and delight.

As my friends stood in the lunch line for cafeteria pudding cups and rectangle pizza slices, I would approach with all of my prepared, preserved, pre-portioned, and preposterous lunch items already arranged on my blue plastic tray. The lunch lady, Miss Nell, knew the routine. She'd reach across the steamy divide for my tray and take it to the stainless-steel recesses of the school's kitchen to rehydrate my main course by covering it with boiling water. We knew this worked better than microwaving, which had once melted a reconstituted burger patty directly onto its little plastic tray, rendering it inedible. That was fine by me. It was a great day, in fact, because she replaced that miserable hockey puck with the fish sticks everyone else was eating.

I carried my tray gingerly back to my lunch table so as not to spill the rehydrating meat juice, since my dry hamburger had to sit in the water for three minutes as it stewed back to life. It was a bit of a tasteless miracle! There it sat in my lunchbox all morning, having been unrefrigerated since leaving the factory (or evil

---

* They all look like Jillian Michaels.

scientist's lair) where it had been produced and packaged, stiff as Styrofoam, into its form-fitting white tray. It looked like a specimen sponge from biology class. But with a hot watery rebirth it bloomed into a somewhat beef-adjacent patty ready for consumption, not enjoyment. The bun came vacuum packed with a shelf life of something like three hundred years. I was hungry enough that it didn't matter.

I am still flabbergasted by the fact that while I was on Nutrisystem, our fridge was so much emptier and our pantry so much fuller. You know you're on a good diet when you don't have to refrigerate anything you eat! Surely, that's a healthful lifestyle choice, especially for a growing teen body!

I do not blame my parents here, as they were doing their best to love me. In their minds, this meant simultaneously feeding me and trying to make me smaller. Sadly, these two goals always cancel themselves out in terms of providing for a child's actual wellbeing.[1] But, to them, Nutrisystem's promises looked like my salvation.

They feared my fatness as a reaper who would steal my future. They imagined I would be unhealthy, unmarried, and underemployed all due to my size. I would suffer stigma and shame. They believed this because they felt stigma and shame in their own fat bodies. They were trying to save me from their own fate. It was misdirected love that started me dieting at five and paid for me to join my first commercial weight-loss regimen at eight. I was growing bigger and bigger, despite all the restrictions. Or, actually, because of all the restrictions.[2] It was desperation that eventually led them to preservative-soaked, water-logged, ridiculously unrealistic diet foods as a potential cure. If tasteless food was the price my family had to pay for my weight loss, so be it. And what a price it was. Nutrisystem costs much more than school lunches would have.

I understood all of this as a kid. And it terrified me. I actually *must be* dying for so much attention and money and time to be focused on making me thinner. I felt fine, but surely that was just masking the diabetes, cancer, heart disease lurking somewhere in my tween frame. It made me strive to outrun my fatness. Not literally, of course. I didn't want to suffer the shame of being the fat girl on the soccer team, and neither did my parents. The uniforms only went up to a certain size anyway. We all knew that if I could just be smaller, just eat "right," I'd gain access to that whole other world of childhood, the "normal" world where kids run and don't get sweaty, eat square pizza and don't have to rehydrate their hamburgers, and aren't an embarrassment to their families.

Back in the school lunchroom, Miss Nell, a very large woman in her own right, helped me every single day. She was kind, as discreet as possible. She understood that I was mortified. I didn't want to ask for this personalized rehydration service any more than she wanted to offer it. Occasionally, she would slip onto my tray an unsanctioned vanilla pudding, my favorite, which I would savor. Surely any calories my parents didn't know I ate weren't *actually* consumed. I was following their diet plan perfectly, at least according to my food diary.

Mama and I would review each other's food diaries in the evenings, an accounting of every morsel eaten, as a means of talking through our days with one another, but also with an ever-vigilant eye toward improvement. I learned that she ate French fries at the bowling alley, a grave transgression. "Well, I guess it evens out. Bowling is exercise," I offered her in absolution, never, ever fessing up to the pudding.

CHAPTER 15:

GOD BECOMES FLESH

Whenever fat activists speak up, we're often ridiculed for "glorifying ob*sity." By this phrase, people mean that fat activists are lifting up fatness as good when it's so clearly bad, vile, embarrassing, [*insert additional vitriol here*]. To glorify ob*sity is laughable, maddening, or even dangerous to those who understand fatness the way our prevalent American culture invites us to. But we've spent some time now looking at the paper tiger that is the "ob*sity epidemic." So, yes, I'm glorifying ob*sity. Guilty as charged.

It's time to glorify ob*sity because bodies like mine should be deemed holy.

I've never been able to reconcile my supposed "badness" as a fat person with the "goodness" of my self-understanding as a child of God. I have always believed in my own "fearfully and wonderfully made-ness" as much as anyone else's, and this necessarily means all of me. Even the fleshy wings of my arms, my soft belly, and ample, dimpled backside. As a Christian minister in the progressive United Church of Christ tradition, how can I preach the unconditional love of God, the radical hospitality of Jesus, and the movement of the Holy Spirit in all flesh but not include my own fat body? How can I readily, through my preaching and activism, challenge the *status quo* marginalization of people by racism, patriarchy, ableism, and homophobia but never question whether their corollaries sizeism and healthism are similar marginalizations at work in the anti-fat hatred that society spews every day?

If fat people are holy, *really holy*—every chin, roll, and jiggle— what would that mean? What would it mean to truly see fat bodies as venerable, worthy bodies, just as they are? Bodies in which the sacred resides not as an afterthought but because fat is an equally valid *imago Dei*? What would it be like to imagine God enrobed in mounds of sacred, fleshy goodness?

Christianity does, in fact, enflesh its deity each and every Christmas Day. On this day, the Christian story goes, God was born on earth in the form of a human baby. This is known by theologians as the "Incarnation of God." The word "incarnation" shares the same Latin root as the words "carnal" and "carnivorous." God taking on flesh.

God comes to earth as a baby lying in a manger. It's a story we Christians celebrate but also take for granted. We may not think about the Incarnation as anything more than a theological underpinning for the Christmas holidays, something mentioned in a festive call to worship and then dropped until next year. But what does the Incarnation really mean for human bodies? What does it mean for God to be "born to us," to choose us, to choose humanity's flesh and blood and bone in which to dwell? The reasonable corollary is that our human bodies, frail and fractured as they are, can somehow also hold divinity in its purest form.

Think about that. A central tenet of Christianity is the idea that the single most divine, powerful entity in the whole universe takes on human flesh, by choice.[1] At Christmas God chose to eat, and walk, and feel the pain of a scraped knee. God chose to have stomachaches, and broken hearts, and anxiety, and all the things that Jesus surely must have felt if he was truly human, one of us, God with us.

This act of an indwelling God validates all of our very humanity with divinity, and not just the modest parts, the pure parts, or the parts we share in polite company. Just as in the Genesis acts of Creation itself, when God called all things good, so does the Christmas Incarnation tell us something about our bodies bearing within them enough goodness to play host to God.

Wow. Except, I don't always feel like my body is a worthy home for God. Some of this is the anti-fatness cultural narrative under which I've lived my entire life. Some of it is the sense of imperfection marketed to me by the diet and beauty industries. And sometimes it's just the frustrating aches of aging, a suddenly sore back from picking up an errant sock the wrong way. Whatever way it comes, my body shame is a more constant companion than it should be. It's times like this that I think: how in the world could *this* flesh be the indwelling place of God? And if I wonder this about myself, maybe you wonder this about yourself, too.

Christianity is an incarnational religion in which deity comes to live among us in the form of a human body. From the beginning, this has been a problem with which the pious must contend: our bodies are both corruptible and our only source of revelation. *Any understanding we have comes from the experience of embodied living.* And yet we live in bodies that ache and lust and hunger. This is what it means to be human, to be a creaturely part of Creation.

We often feel we are at fault when our bodies become sick or painful. We live in a culture where ill-health is understood to be a personal moral failure. That's why we feel ashamed by a new diagnosis, wondering if we could have avoided it with "better" behavior. It's why we speculate about the "lifestyle choices" of the person with lung cancer and are shocked if they never smoked. Or we mentally link a woman's miscarriage and fertility issues to her size, placing blame.

We are embarrassed for those whose bodies don't fit into "norms" of health and beauty as well as ours do. Yet many (or perhaps most) of us also don't like looking at ourselves in the mirror because of all the ways our *own* bodies don't feel worthy. We turn away from and isolate disabled bodies, forgetting that we are all, at all times, one accident, one fall, one pandemic away from our own disability. All of these actions are functions of a culture that denigrates disorderly flesh, that demands we control ourselves and assumes we can, and that moralizes illness as a personal consequence of negative behaviors.

But these bodies of ours are naturally precarious things. They change over time. They age and hurt and die. But I think this is *exactly why* God chose a human body as the vehicle for God's love to come into the world that first Christmas Day. God could have chosen any form God wanted to show the world God's love, to bring us God's light. And God chose to be a baby. Born in a manger. Far away from home. Precarity upon precarity upon precarity.

Its improbability *is* the miracle. Its surprise is the shock of a God who comes to us and then asks to be held, and rocked, and changed, and fed. Mary was asked to tend to God's body in the form of Jesus on that first Christmas Day. And we who follow Jesus are asked to tend to God's body now, to be God's church, to seek the continuation and culmination of God's story on the earth. This is necessarily an embodied task. To do this we must intertwine our own precarious flesh with the precarious flesh of all people, and with all of Creation. We must recognize that God resides in our bodies, and in bodies that look nothing like our own, and treat all bodies with the dignity they deserve.

We are taught by wellness culture to live as though our bodies are autonomous, self-determined things, purely of our own making. The gospel of fat liberation reminds us that we are all a part of God's one big, fat body, the church. It reminds us that we are a collective and interconnected people. With every act of human kindness, with every work of justice, my precarity is made less precarious through its relationship with others. The Incarnation is what makes us powerful agents of collective hope in a world that would sell us only individual freedom.

This is the good news of Christmas Day, the day when God comes to earth first at Bethlehem and in every place thereafter: our fleshy precarity makes us no less worthy of the indwelling of God, but makes us powerful agents of hope. Hope that God's presence within us, within everyone, is a kinship of good bodies, all of us being worthy of dignity and care. Just because Jesus was a man doesn't mean my female body is any less a vessel for divinity. Just because he died young doesn't mean elders can't feel the power of God within their aging bodies.

Disabled bodies, bodies of every hue and size, bodies that lack the resources to shower regularly, bodies that vibrate with pain—these are the bodies where God makes God's home on earth. My body. And your body. God is there, with us. For through the life and ministry and death and resurrection of Jesus, God's spirit was poured out on *all* flesh, not just some flesh.

Every Christmas the Christian church should be reminded of that intimate presence of God in our very bodies. In our creaking bodies. In our aging bodies. In the bodies we keep under heating pads and ice packs. These very bodies of ours are sacred, and good, and enough of a home for the God of the universe.

And if God indeed lives inside all of us, our challenge is to remember this as we encounter others, especially those whose bodies don't look like our own. We must remember that they are equally as worthy of God's incarnation as we are, and that God resides in their bodies, as well. And so, we must work for their dignity just like we would work for our own, until God's reign of justice and peace becomes fully known and realized.

So, hear these words from the beginning of the Gospel of John, and try to listen with your whole bodies:

In the beginning was the Word, and the Word was with God, and the Word was God. He was with God in the beginning. Through him all things were made; without him nothing was made that has been made. In him was

life, and that life was the light of all [humanity]. The light shines in the darkness, and the darkness has not overcome it . . . **The Word became flesh and made his dwelling among us.** We have seen his glory, the glory of the one and only Son, who came from [his heavenly Parent], full of grace and truth.
–John 1:1–5 & 14, New International Version

God breaks into our precious, precarious humanity and finds a home there. This is our incarnational faith. Therefore, let us never doubt that all flesh is, indeed, glorious.

CHAPTER 16:

EMBRACING THE GOSPEL OF FAT LIBERATION EVEN WHEN WE DON'T FEEL IT

The difficult truth is: there is real ambiguity in being fat. I'm several years into my fat acceptance journey. I have come to appreciate the feel and look of soft, fat bodies that are as big and even bigger than mine. I have pride in my fat identity, claim it, and use it to promote the cause of fat acceptance. But I still do not love my fat body as much as I should. At best I have moments of great proximity. It's just plain difficult to live large in a world that is made for the small. It's a daily chore to dismantle my own internalized anti-fat bias and a lifetime of body shame. This truth makes me eternally grateful for my wonderful therapist.

The work of fat liberation is urgent and cannot wait for me to hashtag truly love my upper-arm jiggle. Focusing inward is a sure way to stymie any movement toward societal fat activism and liberative change over and over again. After all, fat liberation is a collective, not just individual, struggle.

Charlotte Cooper speaks of the transgender community using "embodied ambivalence" as a starting place to develop their liberationist strategies.[1] Trans folks can have complicated relationships with their bodies as they live into their most authentic selves within a society that demands specific gender performance. There are both internal and external pressures on trans folks to conform in ways that are limited by binary gender spectrum expectations. One trans essayist named Denny describes her experience with her body saying, "I've never felt at peace with my appearance. Sometimes my desire to be seen can be confusing; I barely have a solid grasp on what I look like, especially to other people. How I feel about myself is nearly always about other people."[2]

Trans and fat activisms align at the point of standing in solidarity against societal hatred for any physical expression outside of the "norm."[3] Cooper points to the work of trans activist Kelli Dunham, who advises that one does not have to love one's own body in order to take care of it and demand its liberation.[4] This is a vitally important point to translate into the fat liberation movement so I will reiterate it again. *One does not have to love one's own body in order to take care of it and demand its liberation.*

Ultimately, the invitation to speak up for the cause of fat liberation even when we don't feel good about our own bodies is an invitation to agency rather than apathy. Internalized weight stigma can lessen fat people's sense of agency,[5] making us feel incapable or unworthy of self-advocacy. Already thoroughly shamed by the culture of anti-fat bias around us, we can't imagine drawing any more attention to our fatness by speaking up for ourselves or others.

I get it. I used to laugh at fat jokes, too, and I sat idly by while colleagues discussed the "badness" of their lunch choices. I dutifully listened to my doctor's salvo of diet tips even when my presenting illness, an earache, had nothing to do with my weight. I promised her I would "do better," and my shame was reinforced when I never could. I watched *The Biggest Loser*, jealous of the contestants' weight loss rather than angered by the physical abuse they were experiencing for the sake of TV ratings.[6] I did these things unconsciously. But deep down, I did these things to prove that I understood fatness to be a negative, unwanted feature. I did this to fit in with the culture even as I stood so obviously apart from it. This is known in fat activist circles as playing the "good fatty," and it is a form of fat respectability politics that tries to mitigate fat oppression by being "in" on the joke.[7] Casual anti-fat hate is a constant barrage, and so it feels daunting to try to make any difference at all. Playing along becomes the path of least resistance, but it's a numbing way to live.

Slowly, over time, I've found that by claiming space, speaking up, and naming anti-fatness for what it is when I experience it, I have grown in confidence as well as agency. I now know that I can effect change, that my fat body is worthy of advocacy, and that I can resist society's anti-fatness even when I still sometimes feel its internal sting. This change has been literally lifesaving. Claiming agency is a hallmark of what it means to welcome a gospel of fat liberation, to build Fat Church.

Let me offer one small example. I have begun unapologetically asking for belt extenders when I fly on airplanes. For years I faked buckling up, tucking the ends of the seatbelt under my shirt to avoid the awkwardness of not fitting in. One time I fell asleep on a long flight and my belt slid off my lap and into the aisle. The flight attendant paused at my seat, woke me up, and gently admonished, "please buckle up," hovering there until I did so. I spent a few graceless seconds trying to pull and prod the belt around my ample waist to no avail other than a growing sheen of nervous sweat. Clearly annoyed, the flight attendant yelled across the quiet plane to her counterpart toward the front, "We need a belt extender for 18C." People turned to look at me. I was mortified and vowed never to sleep on an airplane again.

The flight attendant was clearly disdainful that I undermined the rules of the plane by not buckling. I'd like to think that she wasn't actively trying to fat shame me, though she might very well have been. Either way, it's telling that my first thought was shame at my own failure. My failure to fit a piece of cloth around me and my own sleepy biology were at fault, not the structural issue of airplanes not being built to accommodate people my size. Flying while fat is a harrowing experience,[8] especially as airlines intentionally shrink their seats to maximize their profits.[9]

Traveling frequently for work, my anxiety around flights grew and grew until a day when I was so tired that the thought of not sleeping on the plane outweighed my fat shame. As soon as I stepped into the plane, I quietly asked the first flight attendant I saw, "Can I have a seatbelt extender?" to which he quietly answered, "Sure, sweetie." He handed the extension to me and I slept the flight away, peacefully buckled and giddy at my sudden daring. Since then, I've grown in my ability to speak up for myself. I no longer ask quietly whether I can have a belt extension. Instead, it's a full-throated, "I need a belt extender, please." I name my need and it's always given. Sometimes, when a flight attendant hands me the extension discreetly, I unfurl it in full sight, a visual dare to anyone who would try to make me feel embarrassed by my size.

Seat belt extenders were my starting place. Now I ask for a new chair in restaurants if the one I'm guided to looks paltry for my big frame. I leave the restaurant if they can't give me one, rather than suffering through my meal. I speak up when friends engage in diet talk around me, inviting them to weight-neutral expressions like "I need to move more" as opposed to "I need to lose weight." I sing-song the words "casual fatphobiaaaaa" out loud while I'm watching TV or movies at home, just to mark how many, many times such messages cross my screen. I use free stock images of happy fat people in my presentations[10] and include fat representation in conversations about human diversities in my workplace. I ask people to move over on the bus. I don't shy away from fitting myself onto shared public benches. I read fat activist scholarship every day. I give fat-positive books to those who offer me unsolicited diet advice. I preach on the goodness of all bodies, and I include sizeism and healthism in conversations about systemic oppression. I have changed my social media follows on all platforms to center bodies my size and bigger so I can see fat people thriving daily. And I block every diet or wellness advertisement I encounter, which all-too-conveniently began to rise in my feeds once I added more fat-positive accounts. I can't tell you the joy of liberally reporting all the ubiquitous Noom ads as offensive. It's a small step toward interrupting injustice. Take that, algorithm.

Sometimes it feels like these small, individual disruptions are hardly enough to make a difference in the world. But just like active bystanders can make a difference by calling out racism when they see it, the actions we take to disrupt and correct anti-fatness matter, no matter how small they are. Fat activism typically begins at the individual level, with fat people and their allies shifting their language, their thoughts, and the physical infrastructure in their everyday lives in small ways. If ever this individual activism feels inadequate, there are plenty of opportunities for collective work by joining with fat collectives and organizations that work toward fat acceptance in wider society.

I have taken on my new fat activist habits while still feeling that familiar ambiguity toward my own body. A gospel of fat liberation does not need us to love our bodies; however, *we must act as if we do.* This good news allows me to act on days when I feel strong in my fat pride, and to act on days when society is getting the best of me. Those difficult days are perhaps when I need to claim my agency the most, emboldened not by how I feel about myself but by my unwavering faith in God's good news of body liberation for all.

My body is being judged everywhere I go, a truth that makes my actions important and visible. When I make space for myself, I make space for the other fat people around me. When I point out casual anti-fatness, sizeism, and healthism, I make it visible and harder to replicate thoughtlessly. Even when I feel apathetic about my own worthiness, and cannot fight for myself, I can take up the struggle on behalf of others similarly suffering. My oppression is bound up with yours, and vice versa. Such is the work of social justice. Such is the work of building Fat Church together. And perhaps, when we stand up on behalf of one another, the collective net of care will help us all.

CHAPTER 17:

NEVER LEAVING PARADISE

She's standing there naked as the day she was born, which was just three years ago. Little pumpkin rump of a booty proudly up in the air, hands on the ground, she's wiggling everything she's got in an A-frame of uninhibited joy. Cora's mom, a dear friend, has gone to take something off the stove, leaving open, with its camera on, the laptop on which we've been Zooming our long-distance hellos. Cora's not one to let an audience go to waste. I'm treated to the giddy show of my lifetime. We belly laugh together.

As I look at her in the throes of three-year-old glory, I realize that she's the same age I was when I first became conscious of my body's bigness. My first inkling that I was fat was being told I could not wear the two-piece, frilly, Strawberry Shortcake-themed bathing suit of my dreams the summer of my third year due to the prominence of my protruding toddler tummy. A one-piece was much more suitable. I remember choosing not to be a Brownie[1] like my friends because by second grade I fully understood that I looked "bigger" with a tucked-in shirt, and there was no provision for customizing the uniform toward a more flattering silhouette. When I came home proud of being sat front-and-center in my third-grade class photo, my Mama reacted as if I had been the victim of a cruel joke. Clearly a head taller and several inches wider than my peers, the teachers should have known better; big girls should always be in the back row.

Looking at Cora slap her belly, loving its reverb, I wonder about her future. I know that her Mama will protect her fiercely, but the culture is so, so loud with messages that Cora is sure to hear them. Whether she grows up to be larger or smaller doesn't really matter. The messages are not about reality but self-doubt, anyway.

But, here in this space, well, it might as well be Eden before the Fall. She has not yet eaten of the knowledge that her body even *could* be ashamed. The apple is still on the tree, unbitten. Her nakedness is as comfortable to her as any outfit. When she is clothed, I know that she picks for herself mismatched fashions of bright, clashing pride. Whatever is comfortable or suits her mood. Her green dress does not go with her baby blue shoes. Let's never tell her this.

Her body is completely hers. I wonder how long it will stay that way. I wonder if we could fix the world so it would be hers forever. Wouldn't that be Paradise?

The First Creation Story

In chapter 12, we discussed the Garden of Eden, this paradise of God's good Creation that was supposedly ended for all humankind with Eve's one ruinous bite. She was cast out alongside Adam into a world of shame, pain, and toil. Therefore, woman, she who was made from Adam's rib, has always been understood in traditional Christian circles as a lusty trouble in need of external control. Patriarchal society was shaped on this foundation: women cannot be trusted, and especially not their appetites. Look at where they got us in the first place.

A careful reader of chapter 12's discussion of the Genesis story might remember that I mentioned this was the *second* Creation narrative in our scriptures, and this is true. There is a first one, an earlier one, an alternative one. One that is hiding in plain sight.

Yes, our Bible begins with a contradiction. There are *two different Creation narratives* in the book of Genesis, one placed right after the other presumably for both our convenience and consternation. This obviously competing mythos doesn't get a lot of play in many Christian churches, and some readers may be checking their Bibles right now to make sure I'm not making this up. But they're both there. They are distinct, and, most importantly, they offer two very different views of womanhood.

The *first* Creation narrative, Genesis 1:26–2:3, goes like this:

> Then God said, "Let us make mankind in our image, in our likeness, so that they may rule over the fish in the sea and the birds in the sky, over the livestock and all the wild animals, and over all the creatures that move along the ground." So God created mankind in God's own image, in the image of God, God created them; male and female God created them. God blessed them and said to them, "Be fruitful and increase in number; fill the earth and subdue it. Rule over the fish in the sea and the birds in the sky and over every living creature that moves on the ground." Then God said, "I give you every seed-bearing plant on the face of the whole earth and every tree that has fruit with seed in it. They will be yours for food. And to all the beasts of the earth and all the birds in the sky and all the creatures that move along the ground—everything that has the breath of life in it—I give every green plant for food." And it was so. God saw all that God had made, and it was very good. And there was evening, and there was morning—the sixth day.

> Thus the heavens and the earth were completed in all their vast array. By the seventh day God had finished the work God had been doing; so on the seventh day God rested from all God's work. Then God blessed the seventh day and made it holy, because on it God rested from all the work of creating that God had done.

Such a difference, right? Notice that both male and female* are created in God's image, simultaneously. Both are blessed. Both

---

* Sorry about the binary. Of course, we have a much wider understanding of gender identity and expression now and that's wonderful.

are invited to "be fruitful and multiply." Both are invited to tend to Creation. It is egalitarianism, not complementarianism,[2] that is at work here. A cooperation and a shared responsibility. Equally shared dignity, as well. Tellingly, this narrative does not seem to fit with the second Creation narrative, which starts over from the beginning in Genesis 2:4 as if this first Creation description was just a feminist fever dream.

It's the second Creation narrative that leads into the story of the Fall. It's the second Creation narrative that has God create woman *out of* man, expressly to be his helpmate. It's the second Creation narrative that has *Adam* name Eve, not God. It's the second Creation narrative that then leads toward its intended purpose: to make sure everyone reading the scriptures knows anything bad in the whole wide world, well, that was *her* fault. The original sin of Eve removed humanity from Paradise, and here we all still are.

But what if the second Creation narrative was an addition aimed, at least in part, at explaining why women and their dangerous appetites shouldn't be trusted? What if God's intention for humanity was fully realized in the first Creation story, not the second one? Imagine the difference for women, bodies, and Earth-care if the historic church had focused on a narrative of earthly *goodness* instead of the second Creation story's original *sinfulness*.[3] Imagine a church committed in word and action to continuing the first Creation story—God's good paradise made real here on earth— everyone equally yoked to God, to one another, and to all of good Creation. What if that's actually how it started?

The Church As a Vision of Paradise

Theologians Rita Nakashima Brock and Rebecca Ann Parker wrote the most remarkable book about the fact that, for the first thousand years of the church, it was the image of Paradise, not the image of the Cross, that was the central symbol of Christianity. They say:

As we visited ancient sites, consulted with art historians, and read ancient texts, we stepped back, astonished at the weight of the reality: Jesus's dead body was just not there. We could not find it in the catacombs or Rome's early churches, in Istanbul's great sixth-century cathedral Hagia Sophia, in the monastery churches in northeastern Turkey, or in Ravenna's mosaics. And as we realized that the Crucifixion was absent, we began to pay attention to what was present in early Christian art.

Paradise, we realized, was the dominant image of early Christian sanctuaries. And to our surprise and delight, we discovered that early Christian paradise was something other than "heaven" or the afterlife. In the early church, paradise—first and foremost—was this world, permeated and blessed by the Spirit of God.[4]

In *Saving Paradise: How Christianity Traded Love for this World for Crucifixion and Empire*, Nakashima Brock and Parker argue that the entire life of Jesus, his miraculous healings, his abundant hospitality, his passion, and his resurrection—these things were about bringing life in Paradise to earth once again, not redemptive suffering. They write:

Jesus shows ethical grace in action: love and generosity in community, care for all who have need, healing of the sick, appreciation for life, confrontation with the powers of injustice and exploitation, and advocacy for freedom of the imprisoned . . . In John's Gospel he says, "I came that they may have life, and have it abundantly" (10:10), and he speaks frequently of the promise of "eternal life" to his disciples. The Gospel defines three dimensions of this eternal life: knowing God; receiving the one sent by God to proclaim abundant life to all; and loving each other as he had loved them. Eternal life, in all three meanings, relates to how life is lived on earth. The concrete acts of care Jesus has shown his disciples are the key to eternal life. By following his example of love, the disciples enter eternal life now. Eternal life is thus much more than a hope for postmortem life: it is earthly existence grounded in ethical grace.[5]

According to these theologians, Jesus's "ethical grace," not his crucifixion, became central to the practices of his earliest followers. They attempted to create communities of human flourishing that flattened social hierarchies and the oppressions of empire. And this is why the early Christian church grew! Holy dinner parties! The early church gathered people who had no cultural business fraternizing with one another, save for their shared belief in a new Paradise they were building together here on earth, and it fed them. This was embodied spiritual practice.

The early imagery of the Christian church was filled with representations of life lived abundantly. They often showed lavish depictions of the foods found in Jesus's miracles:

In the Christian catacombs of Rome, images of the loaves and fish are frequent motifs. Large baskets of bread and platters of fish are set around a table with seven people enjoying the food. One delightful image in the Priscilla catacombs shows a table of women. In another, an inscription says the women call, "Bring it warm!" The early church framed its most important ritual meal as this act of feeding. They called it the Eucharist, the Great Thanksgiving.[6]

Christianity was a church built in the fleshiest of ways, one shared meal at a time. It concerned itself with bodies, following Jesus's lead as it eschewed social hierarchies, healed, and fed. This was its attempt to realize God's Paradise here on earth.

What Was Paradise Like?

The Christian Bible's earliest translations, the Greek Septuagint and the Latin Vulgate, translate the Garden of Eden differently than we do. In the Septuagint, it is *paradeisos truphes*, literally "luxurious paradise"; in the Vulgate it's even better, *paradisum voluptatis*, "pleasure paradise."[7] The early Christian church's idea of Eden was not ascetic niceties where Adam and Eve sat around all day considering the majesty of God. They lived it! Eden was full of bodily pleasures, presumably things like eating, sleeping, movement, sex, and playful interactions with the glorious nature around them. It was a voluptuous way of living.

The emphasis on "original sin," which arose alongside "crucifixion-centered Christianity,"[8] bound up the idea of bodily pleasure with the Eve-induced "Fall," rendering flesh no longer innocent but in need of strict control. Conveniently, this shift also allowed the church a great deal of societal power as arbiter of heaven and what constituted "Christian living." By naming what behaviors and people were worthy of salvation, narratives of self-restraint, asceticism, and individual concern for the soul became the norm, while the body—that good gift and source of all human revelation—became no longer a direct line to God but arbitrated by the church. In this way, any craving, lust, or pleasure became suspect.

In much of today's American society, diet culture is even more influential than the church is. The Religion of Thinness is now writing our rules of living, our narratives of self-restraint, asceticism, and individual concern for "salvation" in the form of permanent health, flawless beauty, and ever-lasting vigor.

While the body is no longer understood to be "enough" without unattainable perfection.

We Never Left the Garden

There is a curious fifteenth-century painting by early surrealist Hieronymus Bosch called *The Garden of Earthly Delights*. It is a masterpiece. I remember this work capturing my imagination in my college art history class and my professor's description of it as "a depiction of Eden after the Fall." But is it?

The popular interpretation[9] of *The Garden of Earthly Delights* is that Bosch, a piously Christian man, wanted to show "a debauched world" between the other two paintings that share its triptych.[10] The painting to the right of the three is Bosch's depiction of Creation, showing Adam and Eve with God and the animals in Eden, a calm and pastoral scene. On the left of the triptych is a lewd vision of Hell with demons literally eating and excreting humans, and all manner of human-animal hybrid tortures for the unsaved. But stuck in-between Paradise and Hell is the largest painting, crowded with strange earthly pleasures.

In Bosch's *Garden,* people feast on strawberries and pomegranates as large as themselves. Birds feed humans berries from their beaks. People canoodle while hidden inside mussel shells. Men ride wild boars, bears, and unicorns in a great stampede to the delight of dozens of bathing women nearby, some of whom balance apples on their heads. Everyone is naked, frolicking, and downright goofing off. One cheeky guy puts flowers between his friend's bum. It's a wild scene, no doubt, which many have interpreted (in light of Bosch's Christian piety) as a negative "unnatural" depiction of a depraved world. And if one views *The Garden of Earthly Delights* from the modern-day assumption that Christianity would deem bodily pleasures a "fallen" trait, then it's certainly a lascivious monstrosity. But the colors are vibrant. The people look happy. The scene is chaotic but strangely benevolent. Could there be another interpretation?

Art historian Hans Belting, in his book on *The Garden of Earthly Delights*, offers an alternative interpretation to the scene, one equally as faithful to Bosch's Christian devotion and to the sensibilities of the time. After all, *The Garden of Earthly Delights* was commissioned for the altar of a prominent government official, which means the painting would have been on public display and even visited by dignitaries of other countries within Renaissance Europe.[11] Neither patron nor artist would have wanted to stir the ire of the church.

Belting claims that *The Garden of Earthly Delights* depicts an alternative form of earthly Paradise, one untouched by the Fall. He says:

> The Paradise we are shown here is not the heavenly
> Paradise where the good are welcomed at the end of their
> days, but offers an innocent view of an earthly Paradise
> from which man and woman were never expelled and so
> they need not be judged.[12]

The theme of God's "last judgment" of the earth was popular among artists of the era, who were often commissioned by churches or faithful patrons to depict Christian themes. In fact, Bosch himself had painted another work entitled *The Last Judgment* some years prior. In that triptych, God is pictured above the earth, floating on clouds, clearly looking down on the world's fallenness from a heavenly throne. You can practically hear God's tsk, tsk, tsk. However, God is not pictured above the lusty earth scene in *The Garden of Earthly Delights*. This omission, Belting contends, would have been glaringly obvious to any viewers of its day. Bosch was not giving two renderings of the same story.

In *The Garden of Earthly Delights*, Bosch wasn't depicting a fallen world being judged by God but a world without judgment, as if the Fall had never happened. Bosch's work was intended to be a devotional image of Paradise itself. This would make the first of the three panels in the painting a vision of the *first* Creation story from Genesis, *not* the second story depicting the Fall. Bosch meant for the chaotic earthly scene to be one on which Christians could meditate with joy on what life could have been like in Paradise had the Fall never taken place.

Belting says that Bosch was engaging with a popular theological theme of his day—namely, how humans might have lived if there was no such thing as sin. The late Middle Ages were awash in diseases and social unrest. The unity of the Catholic Church had been shattered by the claiming of two simultaneous Popes. It was a time of transitional powers and of human progress, but it was a difficult time. It makes sense that theologians of the day would have spent time imagining Paradise as a pastime. Paradise might be a place of eternal youth, of frivolous embodiments, of pleasures galore. No death or poverty. No injury or war. Belting believes that Bosch's *Garden of Earthly Delights* was, in fact, about delight, and about "portraying a utopian vision on a grand scale."[13]

Seen in this light, all the strange figures, flora, and fauna of the painting appear less vulgar and more playful. Nakedness and togetherness without shame. Touching as feel-good bodily exploration. Eating for pleasure and fun. Even sticking flowers between one's bum cheeks, I guess (something I could totally imagine my nephews having done when they were younger).

I can see the appeal of theologians and artists using their imaginations to conjure up a new way of life so different from their own. This is, in effect, the same kind of work that Fat Church invites us to do. We need to imagine and then build a church that radically reorders society as we know it today, embracing and protecting fat bodies from shame. We need to paint over the image of an angry God, floating above us in the form of the beauty and diet industries, judging every morsel and fleshy roll. We need to take a cue from Bosch and imagine ourselves living our embodiments to their fullest. And we need to remember that we are faithfully living out God's intention—Paradise on earth—the first Creation story—as we do so.

A Fat Church would radically reorder society. A gospel of fat liberation would free all people from the church's history of body shame so eagerly furthered by diet culture.

Just think of it. Without body shame, what might we do with all that collective freedom?

When I look at pictures of myself at three years old, that precious moment before I knew myself to be fat, I wonder what might have been different about my life had I never been the subject of weight stigma. That question haunts me less for my own life (I'm doing just fine) as for the lives of all the children growing up in diet culture today. When children are without shame their bellies are silly and worthy of blowing raspberries. Their bodily comparisons are made with pure curiosity, not judgment. Wouldn't it be great if they could stay that way?

Back on Zoom, my friend has returned and sees Cora dancing naked. I hold my breath. This is the moment it happens. Fat shame arises from moments like this.

"Don't you wish we could move like that," my friend whispers, in awe.

"Naked dance parties all the time," I reply. We laugh together and Cora wiggles luxuriously in response.

Cora, who will tell you that you are naked? It's not going to be me.

Because at the moment, she is blissfully unaware of how her body—merely its size—could someday define her. At the moment she is dancing, naked, but not ashamed, in a paradise of her own body's making.

A READING GUIDE FOR *FAT CHURCH*

The questions in this guide are meant to help readers reflect on what they have learned from the book and to deepen their commitments to fat acceptance and the wider gospel of body liberation. Readers are encouraged to consider the "questions for personal reflection" privately, where there is space to be unflinchingly truthful and vulnerable. The "questions for group discussion" are more suitable for book groups, workshops, and gatherings where people may be less acquainted with one another.

The work of untangling anti-fatness from our lives will never be complete so long as America's cultural weight bias continues. Still, Christians dedicated to social justice can help end the deadly oppression happening to fat bodies, including their own. Spending time in reflection and re-learning is a starting place, which should be followed by individual and collective action toward a Fat Church, communities where God's good news of body liberation is available to all.

Prologue: Welcome to The Party

Questions for Personal Reflection:

- The prologue lists many groups that are all "welcome to the party." Do you find yourself among them? With which groups mentioned do you self-identify and why?

- Did you have any initial gut reactions to the positive use of the word "fat?" If so, what were they like, and why do you think you did?

- The prologue mentions that this is not a self-help book, nor is it a "God loves you just the way you are" book, but rather it is a fat activism book. Here at the outset, what do you imagine that means, and what are you hoping to learn?

Questions for Group Discussion:

- Take some time to express why you are interested in this book. Name any hopes or fears that you bring with you to this group as you read and discuss *Fat Church* together.

- Share with each other which of the many groups listed as "welcome to the party" you identify with and why. Listen intently while each person shares, and notice how people may or may not resonate with multiple groups simultaneously. Are there any groups of people who were not named but who might also benefit from ending fatphobia in the church and wider society?

- The prologue highlights the power of storytelling, specifically how the power of collective stories can bring about deeper understanding and support. As you engage in this discussion group, remember the power of your own story. How might sharing stories in a group like this enhance the process of reading this book and understanding its message?

Chapter 1: A Big Fat Child of God
Questions for Personal Reflection:

- The chapter begins with the author sharing her life-long struggle with internalized fatphobia stemming from a childhood enmeshed in diet culture. What parts of her story, if any, resonate with your own life?

- The author says that the size of her body was less at issue than the many stereotypes given to fat people—things like lazy, ignorant, diseased, and selfish. What attributes do you associate with fatness and fat people? Do you think these stereotypes are true? If you are fat, do they apply to your own body? If you are not fat, do they apply to a fat person who you personally know and admire?

• Do you have shame about any aspect of your body? If so, where did that shame originate? Consider both the personal experiences and external messages that contributed to that shame. Have you used any interventions or products to "improve" this aspect of your body? If so, did they work? What did they cost you in terms of time, money, or energy? How might your life change if your body shame suddenly disappeared?

Questions for Group Discussion:

• In what ways does your body conform or not conform to societal ideas of a "good body"? Where would you place yourself on a scale between body shame and self-acceptance?

• The author describes how naming herself as "fat"—claiming fatness as a permanent marker of her identity rather than a changeable trait—was a huge step in improving her internalized fatphobia and ending diet culture in her life. What do you think? Regardless of your body size, is fatness an identity marker you would want to claim at this point in the reading? Why or why not? Why do you think fat activists find solidarity and power in claiming fatness as a permanent identity?

• The chapter says that, "God's welcoming embrace is large enough for bodies like mine. It does not demand that I shrink into worthiness. My size is not a sin nor is my fatness indicative of a lack of faithfulness." Do you believe this statement to be true? Why or why not?

Chapter 2: The "F" Word

Questions for Personal Reflection:

- Consider the images you see in media (television, magazines and books, social media, streaming services, movies, advertisements). How many positive representations of fat people do you see daily? Do you follow any body positive or fat acceptance folks on social media? If so, what has it been like to see life through their public postings? If not, search for some now and add them to your social media feeds. Notice what it feels like to see fat people on your screens more regularly.

- A common myth held in society is that fat is a problem to be solved, and a sign of weakened willpower in the person who is fat. Have you participated in believing that myth about yourself or others? What does it feel like to have these myths as driving forces in our lives? Who benefits from such myths?

- The chapter asserts that, "The word 'ob*se' was used in literature as a mocking term for fat people for centuries before it suddenly became a medical description of fatness in the mid-twentieth century." Did you have any idea of the origin or true meaning of this word? How have you heard this word used, and what emotional implications has it carried for you, if any? Do you understand why ob*sity is considered a slur in fat activist circles?

Questions for Group Discussion:

- What alternative words for "fat" have you employed during your lifetime? Why did you use them instead of the word "fat"? Why might someone intentionally avoid using the word "fat" to describe themselves or others?

- Ash Nischuck's "Fatness Spectrum" paints a picture of

the wide spectrum of fat bodies—small fats all the way to infinifat. Had you ever heard of such a spectrum? Do you find it helpful in identifying yourself or others? What biases, if any, arise when you picture a body that inhabits each of the points on this spectrum? Why do you think it is foundational to fat activism to center the experiences of superfat and infinifat people?

- For centuries, to say someone was "ob*se" was to assume gluttony as the origin of their fatness. This understanding of fat is still widespread today even though studies have shown fatness to originate from a complex system of biological and social factors rather than personal choice. Why do you think the pervasive notion of the "gluttonous fat person" persists? Who benefits from understanding fat people as problematic failures of thinness? How might the diet industry use the "gluttonous fat person" trope to its advantage?

Chapter 3: Dangerous but Liberative Unlearning
Questions for Personal Reflection:
- The author likens her experiences unlearning what she was taught by diet culture to unlearning what she was taught by white supremacy culture. Both are intentional and emotional lifelong journeys. Have you had the experience of unraveling "truths" that you later learned were not true despite their pervasiveness? Why do systems persist that are foundationally based on inaccurate accounts and biases? What emotions arise when you do this work? Reflect on what supports you might have at your disposal to help you through the emotions that might arise as you read *Fat Church*. Will those supports reinforce your unlearning of diet culture or undermine it? If you do not have supports for

unlearning diet culture, there are many online communities of fat activists who can support you.

- Think about the description of "respectability politics" in this chapter. Have you ever had experiences of shrinking your sense of self or agency in order to "fit in" to a group? If you are fat, have you ever tried to perform respectability by performing "anti-fatness" in some way—for example, moderating what you eat in public, wearing something to "cover up" your fattest parts, talking about what diet you are on to gain positive attention, or critiquing another's body?

Questions for Group Discussion:
- Look at the bulleted list of arguments that will appear in *Fat Church*. Which argument in the list feels the most "extreme" at this point in the reading? Note any emotions that arise as you consider this argument. Keep this argument in mind as you read the rest of the book to determine whether it still feels "extreme" once you have finished reading.

- The author mentions in this chapter that unlearning much of what she was taught about fatness has been intentional and emotional work, and that it has improved both her well-being and social justice advocacy. Have there been times in your life where you had to unlearn something or shift your thinking about something dramatically? Share with the group what that was like for you.

- Did you know that weight-based discrimination is currently legal in forty-nine out of fifty states? Or that doctors can refuse care to patients above a certain size? Even though these statements are backed up by research, do you have any trouble believing them? If so, why do you think that is?

- If you have a story of size discrimination from your own experience that you are willing to share with the group, please do so. If you do not, please listen to and believe the stories you hear. Does what you've heard point to why ending anti-fat bias in society is important?

The Cookout

Questions for Personal Reflection:

- How is fatness understood in the context of your family of origin and/or chosen family? How have those beliefs filtered into your own understanding of fatness? How are fat relatives or acquaintances treated within your family system? Have you ever been treated differently by your family because of your size?

- Draw a picture of you and your family members in a row, paying careful attention to represent everyone's body size from memory. You can use simple ovals of various sizes if you don't draw well. Just do your best to represent everyone by height and weight proximity. If people have gained or lost weight over time, draw them at whatever weight they were when not dieting. If you know your ancestry, feel free to include grandparents or relatives even farther back, if possible. Look at that visual depiction. Once it's drawn, feel free to find pictures to check its accuracy. Is everyone approximately the same body shape? If there is variety, how do you account for their different sizes? How does your body shape compare to those of your family?

- At what age did you become aware of fatness? At what age did you learn of diets aimed at weight loss? Who taught you about these things and for what reason? Has your belief about fatness changed over your lifetime or stayed the same?

Questions for Group Discussion:

- Copious research shows that restrictive dieting from a young age can cause a host of physical and psychological issues, including higher adult weights and depression, and yet Weight Watchers has launched a program for children as young as 8 and bariatric surgery can now be approved for any child who has gone through puberty. Were you or anyone you know placed on restrictive diets as a child? What was that experience like? Have there been lasting effects carried into adulthood, as there were for the author?

- Have you ever thought about or experienced how weight and body image are portrayed differently by society depending on one's gender? Why do you think that is? Do you think that societal anti-fatness is pointed more toward female-identifying people? If so, why?

Chapter 4: The Prevalence of Anti-Fat Bias
Questions for Personal Reflection:

- Anti-fat hatred is prevalent in society and touches both progressive and conservative circles. How do you identify politically? Have you ever considered how your political views intersect with your feelings about fatness? Or, more broadly, how do your political views intersect with your understanding of issues such as body policing, personal responsibility for health, and food access?

- The story of the New Zealand government refusing a woman's immigration due to her size was eye-opening for the author. Have you ever traveled to another country and experienced a different sensibility toward weight? What is the experience of traveling like for you physically? If you are fat, what physical or other accommodations would make travel easier for you?

- When was the last time you spent money on something aimed at helping you lose weight or "improve" your body in any way, and what was it? How much did it cost? If you had that money in your pocket right now, would you spend it the same way again? Why or why not?

Questions for Group Discussion:

- This chapter explores the prevalence of anti-fatness in American society across the political spectrum. Have you seen politicians or public figures critiqued for their fatness as a means of undermining their ideas? Do you think that fat shaming is a fair or effective strategy in politics?

- Bias based on perceived race and weight bias are named in this chapter as the two most common forms of bias in American society. How do these two forms of bias interplay with one another? How are they different from one another?

- Had you previously considered how the "wellness industry" aligns with diet culture or politically aligns with notions of personal responsibility for health? Can you remember any advertisements for wellness brands that explicitly name or imply weight loss as a function of using their products? Does that make their products more or less appealing to consumers, do you think? If they made their sales pitch weight-neutral, do you think it would have the same appeal?

- The endnotes are a helpful resource in this book. The research includes commentary and connections that will enhance the reading. Choose one endnote from the chapters you've read thus far that you would like to share with the group.

Chapter 5: Women, Wasps, and Weight

Questions for Personal Reflection:

- In what ways do you feel personally responsible for your family's health? What measures do you take to support the health of those you love? After considering the adverse effects of weight stigma, could you imagine any of those measures to be more harmful than helpful?

- It can be difficult for those of us enculturated to hate fatness to realize the ways in which that bias was built on the foundations of racism, classism, religious bigotry, and xenophobia. As you encountered this chapter, what emotions arose in you? Were there any sections that were particularly emotional to read?

- C. Everett Koop, the Surgeon General who declared America's first "War on Fat" in 1994, did so after his own twenty-five-pound weight loss. This is an extreme case of the "weight-loss evangelism" that happens around us every day. A friend gifts a diet book to another friend. A coworker gives unsolicited diet advice like, "I cut out the carbs and feel so much better!" A relative says that they are "concerned for the health" of their fat family member. Have you ever been a weight-loss or diet-culture evangelist in one of these ways? If so, how might your actions have been harmful instead of helpful?

Questions for Group Discussion:

- This chapter begins by stating that, historically, "family health was considered women's work, part of managing the home." Do you think this is still true today? Why or why not?

- What historical fact from this chapter has stuck with you the most? Why do you think it stuck with you?

- Body Mass Index (BMI) is widely used to study and treat people of all sizes. It's used as the basis for pricing and receiving medical and life insurance coverage. It's used to categorize people into diagnostic groups of perceived "health." Were you surprised at the racist origins of the BMI, or the fact that it was never meant to be attributed to individual bodies at all? Does this fact change the way you understand the BMI? Do you think the claim that the BMI is "too widely used" is a good excuse for why the BMI has not been removed from medical use? How might the decision to continue using the BMI as a measure of "health" perpetuate harm of fat people and people of color?

- Were you surprised by the ways Protestant church leaders participated in spreading the notion that personal health is one's own responsibility, a moral obligation of living a "good Christian life"? In what ways do you hear that notion of health echoed in churches today?

Chapter 6: The Polarizing Figure of the Unrepentant Fat Woman

Questions for Personal Reflection:

- Read again the initial description of the unrepentant fat woman at the start of this chapter. Note the feelings that arise in you while reading it. Do you feel envious of this woman? Do you pity her? Are you scared of her or repulsed by her? Are you picturing someone you've seen in public who fits her description, or perhaps a fat celebrity? Notice how you feel reading this description at this point in the book. Make a note to reread it at the end of the book and see whether your feelings have changed toward this woman at all.

- Are there particular times of the year when you feel better or worse about your body? What is happening during those seasons to make you feel that way? Make a chart of the times of the year when diet culture arises in media and marketing in particularly loud ways. Does this chart align at all with how you feel about your own body?

- The chapter mentions how the problematic words "morbid ob*sity" can feel like a death sentence in the hands of the medical profession. It hurts to be understood as mortally endangered by one's own body shape. Have you ever felt like your body was a liability rather than a blessing? If so, how did these feelings lead you to treat your body over time?

Questions for Group Discussion:

- The chapter describes how Michelle Lelwica's "Religion of Thinness" in America has its own liturgical year cycle that has become so ingrained in our culture that we may not even think about it anymore. Read over that cycle description once again together. Consider how America's formal and informal holidays are marketed with regard to food and bodies.

- Is there anything missing from the description of the "Religion of Thinness's" yearly cycle? What about personal events—birthdays, anniversaries, family reunions, vacations? How are food and bodies part of those celebrations?

- Discuss the "body positivity" movement as a group. Have you noticed that more fat people are being used in commercials and advertisements as of late? Representation matters, so this is something to be celebrated! Yet the chapter also names the limitations of the "body positivity" movement, especially how it has been coopted to sell products rather than to end systemic anti-fat discrimination. Do you think this is a fair critique? Why or why not?

• How do you feel when you see fat people in commercials? Do you take notice? Does it make you more or less likely to purchase a certain product, or to look longer at the advertisement? Are you seeing representation of all sizes of fat bodies along the "Fatness Spectrum," or just smaller fat bodies?

The Recipe Box

Questions for Personal Reflection:

• What is your favorite recipe to make or eat that has been passed down from someone you love? How does that food make you feel when you eat it? Think of the best meal you ever ate. What do you remember about it? Why do you think you can remember it still today?

• What were dinners like in the household of your youth? Did you sit at the table together or did everyone fend for themselves? Did a parent cook for you or did you make your own food most of the time? Did you have enough to eat or were you regularly left wanting? How did your guardians approach food? As a joyful blessing? As a troublesome necessity? As a mechanistic way to power body-machines? Do any of these childhood eating memories influence your adult eating patterns still today?

Questions for Group Discussion:

• Consider doing a recipe swap within your group. Each

person should bring a recipe that raises a positive emotion in them—pleasure or delight, a happy memory of someone who once made it, or a positive memory from a particular time eating it. Bring these recipes written out in their original form, and don't worry whether everyone in the group can use each recipe. There may be legitimate dietary restrictions among you such as food allergies or moral obligations (like eating vegan or kosher) that will preclude everyone in the group from using every recipe. That's alright. Every person who feels comfortable should read their recipe aloud, preferably handing out or sending a copy to the other members of the group so they can read along. Then they should share the reason they chose this recipe in particular.

- Listeners should note the variety in the recipes—the different flavors and styles of cooking represented. There are so many foods that bring people positive emotions. When we eat for comfort or joy it may be the best thing we could do for ourselves in that moment. Flavors connect us to our loved ones throughout time. And yet "emotional eating" is decried by diet culture. Why do you think that is? Isn't all eating emotional in some ways? Why or why not?

- Everyone's recipe should be valued as something that brings them positive emotion. If you are tempted to comment on any recipe in any negative way, do not do it. Keep that comment to yourself. But do consider the origins of your critique. Are you moralizing some aspect of the recipe as "good" or "bad"? Do you imagine that it's a flavor you wouldn't enjoy? Practice honoring another person's food choices without any judgment. Try to celebrate every recipe for the joy it brings the other person.

Chapter 7: The Way We Understand Fat Is Cultural
Questions for Personal Reflection:

- This chapter invites the reader to claim fatness as a permanent marker of one's identity rather than a temporary state from which diets will save them. How did you feel encountering the research on how diets don't work for long-term weight loss? Do you feel that the diet industry is acting in good faith for the wellness of its customers, or simply trying to make as much money as possible?

- Have you ever felt yourself to be "at war with fat" during your lifetime, either within yourself or in others? How does that language fit with your understanding of fatness now?

- Having read *Fat Church* to this point, have you changed at all in your perception of fatness since page one?

Questions for Group Discussion:

- What is a cultural shift you have witnessed in your lifetime? Do you think that attitudes about fatness might similarly be able to change? What actions would help change the culture of anti-fat hate in America? What benchmarks or metrics would show that weight stigma was ending?

- Read once again J. Eric Oliver's quote at the end of the chapter about his own research into fatness, in which he names three prevailing assumptions about fatness. Have you held any of these assumptions yourself? What other assumptions about fatness do you hold at this point that might need investigating?

- Discuss the calculated movement among diet industry leaders to shift fatness from a body type to a disease in and of itself. Why was this move helpful to their industry? Has this cultural shift influenced your understanding of fatness? Do you consider fatness itself a disease? If so, how might that belief be challenged by the research within this book?

Chapter 8: An Unholy Trinity: The Diet, Beauty, and Medical Industries

Questions for Personal Reflection:

- Are you currently investing your time, energy, or money in any weight-loss regimens? If so, how did reading this chapter make you feel about those efforts?

- If you are currently on a diet or exercise regimen and are seeing "progress" in the form of weight reduction, will you feel like a failure if your weight grows again someday? If so, do you imagine that you will blame yourself and your body for the failure, or might you consider focusing your anger toward the diet industry, which knows its products do not work in the long run? What might it take for you to step off the diet culture hamster wheel for good? Could you imagine never dieting again? If that makes you anxious, why? In what other ways could you spend your time, energy, or money feeling good in the body shape you have?

Questions for Group Discussion:

- Have you noticed diet, exercise, and weight-loss programs recently pivoting their marketing from mechanistic diet regimens to softer words like "health coaching," "body positivity," "mindfulness," and "holistic health," instead of "calorie counting" or "feeling the burn"? Why do you think this shift is happening in diet culture today? What impact do you think it makes on the next generation of people seeking weight loss?

- Sonya Renee Taylor calls the diet industry the "Body Shame Profit Complex." After reading this chapter, do you agree that the diet industry is a self-perpetuating form of capitalism, creating both the products promoting weight loss and the anti-fat hate necessary to sell them? Why or why not?

- The chapter describes how doctors suffer from confirmation bias as readily as the rest of us do, which can lead to treating patients more or less thoroughly depending on the doctor's perception of that person. If you are a minoritized person because of one or more of your identities, have you ever felt stigmatized by your doctor? Did you suspect that this stigma led to lesser care in some way? If you feel comfortable doing so, tell your story to the group. For those who have not had this experience, listen to and believe them.

- Take Harvard's Implicit Association Test (IAT), which is free of charge and located online at: https://implicit.harvard.edu/implicit/takeatest.html. Share with the group your experience of taking the IAT. Did anything surprise you? Did you take any of the other available tests? How did your implicit bias toward fatness compare to any other implicit bias you tested?

- What is your reaction to learning about the Minnesota Starvation Experiment? What do you make of the fact that the caloric understanding of starvation in the experiment (1,600 calories) is the same number of calories promoted by many diets for weight loss still today?

Chapter 9: Big Fat Truths about Ob*sity
Questions for Personal Reflection:
- The research in this chapter shows how weight cycling from restrictive diets is more harmful to one's body than living in

a stable-sized fat body over a lifetime. Was that surprising to learn? How did it make you feel about your own history of dieting, if you have one? Even if you have never dieted, how does this make you feel about the diet industry as a whole?

• If you are not a fat person, or if you have at times in your life been "thin," how did you react to the notion of "thin privilege"? If you have grown fatter or thinner over the course of your lifetime, have you noticed a change in how you are treated by friends, family, strangers, or the medical industry based on your size?

Questions for Group Discussion:

• Look at Harriet Brown's list of ailments that are associated with yo-yo dieting (also known as weight cycling) at the start of this chapter. Do you associate these illnesses with fatness? Why or why not? If researchers know that weight cycling causes harm, and that long-term weight-loss is not possible for most people, why do you think diet culture persists? Why is it that doctors still prescribe weight-loss interventions to patients when they are known not to work, or to actually cause harm? Can you think of any other medical intervention that a doctor would prescribe a patient where the research shows such a high percentage of failure?

• Ob*sity researchers are beginning to publicly decry the weight stigma associated with fatness, understanding the ways it causes ill-health effects in fat people. This is a good thing! However, many of these same ob*sity researchers still manage weight-loss clinics, receive funding from the diet industry, and promote an overall culture of anti-fatness. Do you see this as a conflict of interest? Why or why not?

- If you are fat and a pill existed that reduced a person's size to a medically "normal" BMI and yet had unknown side effects, would you take that pill? Would you encourage the fat people you know to take it? Why or why not?

- Were you surprised to learn how little research goes into treating fat patients for ailments other than ob*sity? Or that pharmaceutical trials rarely factor in body weight variation to their dosing, despite the prevalence of fatness in America? What do you think causes this systemic lack of research on fat people? Do you think this lack of research factors into fat people's overall health outcomes?

- Did the fact that the diet industry was allowed by the Federal Trade Commission (FTC) to be self-regulated surprise you? Would you have agreed with the FTC's decision? Why or why not?

The Parable of The Two Knees

Questions for Personal Reflection:

- Have you ever been denied care by a doctor or other professional because of your body size or weight? Or do you know someone who has? If so, what was that experience like?

- If you have not previously experienced medical weight bias on this level, imagine being the young mother in the story, denied surgery because of your weight. What would that experience be like? How would you feel about yourself? How would you feel about the medical industry?

Questions for Group Discussion:

- Discuss the differences and similarities in these two

women's stories. Now discuss their different healthcare outcomes. Do you believe the inequity in their treatment is justified? Why or why not?

- Fat people are often denied routine treatments and surgeries prescribed to thinner people because doctors demand they lose weight first. Thinking back to what you have learned in the book thus far, why do you think this is? What emotions arise as you consider these inequities in health care that befall people in fat bodies?

- Perhaps you have watched television shows like *My 600-lb Life* where infinifat people are publicly displayed receiving bariatric surgery. Why do you think bariatric surgery is routinely approved for the largest bodies when other surgeries are not?

Chapter 10: The Question of "Health"
Questions for Personal Reflection:

- Spend some time considering the question raised at the start of this chapter: "If you had the choice between your body being a perfectly proportioned example of toned, socially desirable thinness and yet unhealthy, or four-hundred pounds and yet healthy, which would you choose?"

- Many fat people experience the shame of being "concern trolled." This happens when a stranger, friend, or relative offers unsolicited feedback that they are "concerned for the health" of the fat person, often imploring them to lose weight as a performance of "improved health." This is a healthist action rooted in anti-fat bias. Have you ever concern trolled someone or been concern trolled yourself? What was that experience like for you? What did that

experience change for anyone involved? Do you think it
was helpful?

- The chapter reports, "health researchers have found
that, without the promise of losing weight, people are
unmotivated to increase their health behaviors. Most people
are willing to adapt their diets and increase their exercise
only if it means 'they will look better.'" Is this the case for
you? Why or why not?

Questions for Group Discussion:
- How do you define "health"? Are there differences among
you in how you define "health"? Why do you think those
different definitions of "health" exist?

- The chapter claims that, "American culture makes
'health' a primary goal of its citizenry because a person's
wellness presumably translates into their productivity
as a worker and, thereby, their ability to be a consumer."
Health insurance often being tied to one's employment
is an example of this value at work in society. What
other evidence supports or refutes this claim? How does
consumerism intersect with "health" in America?

- Imagine that the "fat gene" could be isolated and doctors
had the ability to turn it off before a person's birth. Would
this be a good thing or a bad thing for society? What would
society gain or lose from the eradication of all fat people?
This same question is being asked about other human
diversities, as well. If doctors could isolate the "gay gene,"
or the "neurodivergent gene," or the "disability gene,"
would you make the same decision about eradication? Why
or why not?

- Had you heard of the concept of "healthism" before? Do you believe that "health" is one of this country's primary moral values? Why do you think that is? Do you think "healthism" stigmatizes those who are not perceived to be "healthy" in American society? If so, how so? Where have you seen examples of healthism or healthist bias in your own experience?

The Carrot

Questions for Personal Reflection:

- Have you ever been to a nutritionist or other food-based wellness professional? What was that experience like? Did your eating habits change while working with them? If so, have you maintained those changes? Why or why not?

- What is the most nutritious meal you can think of? What are its flavors and textures? What would it cost to make or procure? Would you enjoy that meal? How would it make you feel to eat that meal? Consider how you would feel both physically and morally. Would you feel like a "better person" if your food intake always roughly matched that meal? If yes, consider why you would feel that way. In light of what you've read so far, do you think any of the reasons are due to food moralization or internalized fatphobia?

Questions for Group Discussion:

- Do you think the cultural concept of "nutrition" is affected by diet culture in America? If so, how?

- Reflect on your own self-image. Does your self-image change depending on the foods you eat on any given day? If so, how, and do you believe any of that internal narrative stems from fatphobia or diet culture?

- If you had a carrot and an Oreo in front of you right now, which would you eat and why? Would your choice change if you were home alone instead of in a group? If your choice would change, why is that? Have you ever changed your food choices based on the people around you rather than your own internal hunger and pleasure cues? If so, why?

Chapter 11: Disbelief Is a Starting Place
Questions for Personal Reflection:

- Our commitments to social justice movements can wane when we begin to feel discomfort. It takes a great deal of personal effort to dismantle our internalized oppressions and live in a countercultural way. Assimilating back into the patterns and behaviors we are used to is sometimes much easier, but this "return to normal" comes at a price when we've learned what harms these patterns and behaviors cause. ("White fragility" is one example of how people can become defensive of their worldviews and patterns rather than making the effort to change.) Has what you've read in *Fat Church* made you uncomfortable? In what ways? If you have begun to consider enacting a countercultural attitude toward fatness or marginalized bodies in general, how might you withstand the pull back toward assimilation within diet culture? What supports do you need to continue forward on your journey, rather than turning back?

- This chapter references many fat activists and anti-diet-culture researchers. Pull up some of these names online. Look at their social media presence and the books or articles they've written, and get a feel for their voice and general persona. Make note of some who you want to revisit later for a deeper dive into their work.

- Do you resonate with either of the "yeah, but" excuses mentioned in this chapter? Would you add any further "yeah, buts" that are causing you doubt and that need "exorcising" before you can believe in fat acceptance and the gospel of body liberation?

- Do the exercise discussed in this chapter. If you are fat, write out a list of the things that make your life difficult because you are fat. If you are not fat, write out a list of the things you imagine might make life difficult for a fat person. Evaluate your list. Which of these things would no longer be difficult if medicalized diet culture and anti-fat bias went away tomorrow, and if public spaces were accommodating of fat bodies? Which of these things could you help change on your own or by joining with other fat activists?

Questions for Group Discussion:
- The research within this book has outlined some of the myths, outright lies, and problematic corporate behavior of the medical, diet, beauty, and wellness industries that have gone mostly unchecked (or even been celebrated) in American culture. Have any of these realizations been shocking to you? If so, which facts in particular are sticking with you? Is any of what you've read making you rethink participation in diet culture or anti-fat bias in any way? Why or why not?

- Do you think it's fair that straight-sized researchers are believed more readily than fat researchers about anti-fatness? Why do you think that is the case?

Chapter 12: Original Sin, Self-Control, and "Good" Christian Bodies

Questions for Personal Reflection:

- What are the teachings of the church that have influenced how you feel about human bodies? Were you taught that bodies were universally good, abject, or somewhere in-between? Were you taught by the church that certain bodily behaviors were morally sinful or righteous? Were there differences in acceptable behaviors depending on gender, sexuality, or ability? Can you remember particular lessons, sermons, or experiences that reinforced those teachings? Which teachings do you agree with still today and which have you put aside? If you have put any church teachings aside, what made you do so?

- If you identify as female, have you ever felt the modern-day ramifications of the church's patriarchy in your religious or personal life? If so, how?

Questions for Group Discussion:

- This chapter describes the philosophy of "dualism," which suggests things of the body are corrupt while things of the mind/soul are separate from the body and thus more holy. Do you believe this to be true? If so, what has shaped this belief? Do you believe American society functions as if dualism were true? In what ways do you see dualism at work in your everyday life?

- Had you ever heard of "complementarianism" before reading this chapter (the idea that men and women were created differently by God and that women's role is to be a "help-mate" to man)? In what ways do you see that theology still at work in the modern-day Christian church or in wider society?

- The historic Christian church has shaped society in a number of ways. Where do you see the influence of the Christian church in American culture either explicitly or implicitly? Has the church's influence always been toward societal good? If not, where has it been used to promote problematic or even evil things? Give examples as they come to mind.

- If you believe in an afterlife, do you believe our spirits will be embodied there? If so, what is your idea of a "heavenly body," or the body that goes to be with God in some way after death? Do you imagine this heavenly body to be much like bodies here on earth, or would it be "perfected" in some way? If so, how? How might our notions of what bodies are like in the afterlife affect how we see bodies in the here-and-now? What about Christians who live in bodies marginalized by society in some way? Will their bodies change in the afterlife or will societal marginalization change in the afterlife?

The Parable of the Weeds
Questions for Personal Reflection:

- The poet in this parable struggles with the weeds in her garden until the moment when she claims them as wanted rather than problematic. Did this sentiment speak to you in any way? What do you believe the poet was trying to get across with this poem?

- Reflect on the relationship you have had with your body over the course of your lifetime. Have there been times of acceptance, or even pride at your appearance? Have there been times of shame or disgust? What factors contributed to the ways you've felt about your body over the years?

- What part of your body feels most like a weed in the garden to you? Like the poet did for her weeds, might you be able to create another, positive narrative for that part of your body? If you could welcome that part of your body fully, how might your feelings about yourself change? Would any of your behaviors change?

Questions for Group Discussion:

- *Fat Church* contains two parables: the "Parable of the Weeds" and the "Parable of the Two Knees," which was earlier in the book. What is a parable? Why do you think these two parables are included in the book?

- As a group, discuss the message of the "Parable of the Weeds." Take note of the ways each person thinks about the story, especially noting any different interpretations. What lessons can be taken from this parable?

- What do you think "revolutionary hospitality" means in the context of fat acceptance and body liberation? What kinds of ideas or practices would be necessary to enact revolutionary hospitality within one's own life? How about within the Christian church?

Chapter 13: Jesus and the Reluctant Saints of Fat Liberation

Questions for Personal Reflection:

- Consider your personal experience within religious communities during your lifetime. Have you ever experienced fatphobia, food moralizing, or body shaming in any of those communities? If so, what was that like? What impressions did those experiences leave with you about yourself, about that particular religious community, or even about religion in general?

- The chapter describes some of the early writings of the fat rights movement as "unfiltered and deliciously filthy in their disregard for respectability." What do you think this means? Could you imagine any benefit in eschewing "respectability" for "authenticity"? What might the dangers of living authentically be? If you were not concerned with being "respectable" for one whole day, would it change the way you acted, dressed, ate, spoke, or otherwise engaged the world? What wild action might you take if you were bold and shameless enough to do it?

Questions for Group Discussion:

- Had you ever considered how many stories about Jesus from the Christian gospels have to do with food? Why do you think the gospel writers focused so much on Jesus eating with and feeding his disciples?

- Look up an image of the Venus of Willendorf online. This is one of the oldest pieces of art ever uncovered—more than 20,000 years old! She is proof that fat people have existed all throughout history. Jesus would have known some fat people in his day. How do you think Jesus felt about the fat people he encountered? How might he have treated them?

- The author recounts experiencing anti-fatness and weight stigma in churches that were very different from one another both theologically and geographically. What common traits might these churches still have shared? Do you think that these commonalities might have served to uphold these churches' similar cultures of anti-fatness? Why or why not?

- How do you understand the concept of "Fat Church"? What might a religious movement or community rooted in true body liberation be like? How might it impact the wider Christian church or even society?

Chapter 14: Jesus Heals a Woman

Questions for Personal Reflection:

- This chapter uses an imaginative retelling of a gospel story to explore what "healing" might have meant to a fat woman seeking a miracle from Jesus. Did you see yourself reflected in any of the characters of the story—the woman desperately seeking healing, the crowd pressing in to see the spectacle, or those who stood by in judgment of the woman? Did reading this chapter bring up any emotions for you?

- The author implores fat readers to want more than societal assimilation for themselves. What do you think she means by this?

- At the end of this chapter, the author once again makes the case for understanding fatness as a permanent identity marker rather than a disease to be cured. If you are fat, is this an identity you can imagine claiming for yourself at this point in the reading? Why or why not?

Questions for Group Discussion:

- The Christian church has been complicit in deep societal wounds like structural racism. And yet churches are often unwilling to engage in the difficult work necessary for true repentance and healing. Why do you think this is the case? Can you give examples of "sacred bandages" that churches have attempted to place over these deep societal wounds in order to obscure the problem rather than fully address it?

- One of the central points of this chapter is that Jesus's miraculous healings were not only for those individuals he helped but were symbols of the communal healing God intends for wider society. Do you believe this is true? If so, what are some of the ways you think God might want society to heal?

- Assuming the Christian church has a responsibility to help heal the ills of society, especially those in which it has been complicit, where should it start? What steps might the church take to move beyond the "sacred bandage" approach and into deeper exploration of societal wounds? How might the church help bring about the corporate societal healing that Jesus intended?

The Pantry

Questions for Personal Reflection:

- Think back to the experience of eating lunches in the schools of your youth. What was the social dynamic like in the cafeteria? Did you bring your food to school, did you purchase it, or was it provided for you in some other way? Did you have enough to eat? Did you trade food items with friends? Did you make fun of the person whose lunch was "different" in some way? Or was that person you? Have those experiences of communal eating as a young person left any lasting impressions on you?

- Were you ever placed on a diet as a child? If so, was everyone in your household on the same diet? What message did dieting as a child send to you? What are some of the emotions you remember feeling at this time of your life?

- The author remembers thinking as a child, "I must be dying for so much attention and money and time to be focused on making me thinner." *Fat Church* has outlined the diet industry's efforts to shape cultural understandings of fatness from a body shape into a deadly disease. The myth of premature death is part of that effort, and yet this myth persists as a fear for many fat people. Have you ever feared a premature death because of your body size? If so, did this fear change the way you thought about or treated your body?

Questions for Group Discussion:

- Storytelling can be a very powerful tool for building empathy and understanding. If you were to write a story from your life called "The Pantry," what would you say? Give this some thought silently as individuals and then, as you feel comfortable, share with each other your "pantry" stories.

- How do children become exposed to diet culture and weight stigma? Brainstorm as a group at least ten different ways this exposure might happen. Do you think it's possible to shield children from diet culture and weight stigma in America, or is this an inevitable part of growing up in our society? If you believe it's inevitable, what would need to change for it not to be? How might parents push back against the messages of anti-fat hate, healthism, and body shame perpetuated by diet culture?

Chapter 15: God Becomes Flesh
Questions for Personal Reflection:

- The chapter begins with the declaration, "It's time to glorify ob*sity because bodies like mine should be deemed holy." How did you initially react to that statement when you read it? Do you agree with it, or does this statement make you pause in some way?

- Many fat people have had the phrase "your body is a temple" leveled at them as a form of moralizing their body shape as sinful. How might you reclaim the idea that your body is, in fact, a temple for God just the way it is, no matter what your body type or ability, without needing to change in any way? Where in your body do you feel God's presence the most?

- Does an incarnational theology, one in which God chooses to take on human form, make you think differently about your own body or bodies more generally?

Questions for Group Discussion:

- Reflect on the idea of the Incarnation, the choice by God to dwell among us in human form. What do you think that decision says about God? What do you think that decision says about humanity?

- The author writes, "our bodies are both corruptible and our only source of revelation. Any understanding we have [of God, or anything else for that matter] comes from the experience of embodied living." What do you think she means by this? Is this statement true? If so, how might this idea challenge the notion of dualism (that mind/soul is separate somehow from the body) that was explored at the beginning of chapter 12?

- Imagine a time in which fatness is no longer equated with sinfulness. How might society benefit from that change?

- Diet and wellness culture promote the understanding that our bodies are ours alone, autonomous and self-determined. Does this "personal responsibility narrative" still feel valid alongside a theology of Incarnation? How does the idea of "personal responsibility" for one's body alone interact with the notion that all people of the church are collectively the Body of Christ on earth?

Chapter 16: Embracing the Gospel of Fat Liberation Even When We Don't Feel Like It

Questions for Personal Reflection:

- Think about Charlotte Cooper's concept of "embodied ambivalence," a way of demanding dignity and care for one's own body while still having complicated feelings toward it. The work of fat activism would never begin if we all waited for everyone to love every part of themselves. If you are fat, or if you have been enmeshed with diet culture, how might you embrace embodied ambivalence as a strategy to put any personal "body-feelings" aside in favor of unapologetic advocacy against anti-fat hatred?

- The chapter describes the concept of the "good fatty," or the fat person who actively participates in anti-fat rhetoric and self-deprecation in order to prove they understand fatness as a "problem," and thus fit into society. Examples include things like laughing at fat jokes, listening to others' fatphobic rhetoric without pushing back, eating differently in public, and judging others' size in comparison to one's own. If you are fat, have you ever fallen into the trope of the "good fatty" in social situations? Do you think this was helpful behavior? If you were in those situations again, would you change how you behaved? Why or why not?

Questions for Group Discussion:

- Have you ever had the experience of speaking up for yourself or another person against an injustice? Feel free to share stories within the group. How would you describe that experience emotionally? Was the act of speaking up difficult to do? Why or why not?

- The author discusses some small interruptions to fatphobia that she has been trying in her own life. Take a couple minutes for each person to list three small actions they could begin doing right now to resist diet culture and societal anti-fatness. These could be actions within your own life, home, family system, church community, or wider society. After everyone has had a chance to reflect personally, name some of these aloud within the group.

- The chapter ends: "My oppression is bound up with yours, and vice versa. Such is the work of social justice." Reflect as a group on the ways in which this statement is lived out or not lived out in personal relationships, families, the church, and/or wider society.

Chapter 17: Never Leaving Paradise
Questions for Personal Reflection:

- Think of the story of little Cora. Do you remember a time in your life when you were truly free with your body? If so, what was that like? If not, what messages limited your sense of body freedom?

- Encountering diet culture myths and their pervasive reach on American culture can be an emotional endeavor. Has reading *Fat Church* unearthed any emotions within you such as anger, grief, confusion, vindication, relief, shame, frustration, excitement, or remorse? How are you feeling at this point, having read the whole book? Is it an overall positive or negative feeling? Do any of the emotions you feel conflict with one another? What is the next step you plan to take given all you have learned?

Questions for Group Discussion:

- The chapter points out that the Bible begins with a contradiction. It presents two different Creation narratives side-by-side right at the start of the book of Genesis. Had you ever noticed this before in your reading of the Bible? Have you ever heard this contradiction preached or discussed in Bible study? If not, why do you think that is? Does it surprise you that the two Creation narratives are so different from one another? Can you think of any other contradicting messages within the Biblical text? How do you make sense of these contradictions?

- Has Jesus's death on the cross been the central theme of your understanding of Christianity or has Paradise? How might recovering a theology that centers Paradise rather than crucifixion change the church's way of engaging in the world? How might a Paradise-centered theology help the Fat Church cultivate a gospel of body liberation?

- As a group, do an internet search for "Hieronymus Bosch: The Garden of Earthly Delights" and look closely at the center panel of the artwork described in this chapter. What do you make of it? Does the frivolity of the scene seem playful or lascivious to you? Is it somewhere you would like to be (presuming you harbored no body shame)? What is your favorite image in the scene? If Bosch did, indeed, paint this as an "innocent" representation of humanity in Paradise, never having been affected by sin, then what does this say about Bosch's view of human bodies as part of God's good Creation?

- Were you surprised to learn from theologians Nakashima Brock and Parker that the central symbol of Christianity during its first thousand years was Paradise rather than the crucifixion? You can read their book to learn what brought about this change, but do you have any immediate theories? How do you think this change in theological emphasis (from Paradise to the cross) influenced the teachings of the church from that point forward?

- What is the central idea or lesson you will take from *Fat Church*?

ENDNOTES

Section 1: First Things First

1   Michelle M. Lelwica, *The Religion of Thinness: Satisfying the Spiritual Hungers Behind Women's Obsession with Food and Weight* (Carlsbad, CA: Gürze Books, 2010), 78.

Prologue: Welcome to The Party

1   Cecilia Hartley, "Letting Ourselves Go: Making Room for the Fat Body in Feminist Scholarship," in *Bodies Out of Bounds: Fatness and Transgression*, ed. Jana Evans Braziel and Kathleen LeBesco (Berkeley: University of California Press, 2001), 60–73.

2   Charlotte Cooper, *Fat Activism: A Radical Social Movement* (Bristol: HammerOn Press, 2016), 9.

3   "Intersectionality" is a term that legal scholar Kimberlé Crenshaw coined in 1989 to describe how multiple oppressions and privileges exist alongside one another. For example, women often suffer the effects of patriarchy in their lives, but a Black woman experiences the intersection of both racialized oppression and gendered oppression. Someone who is disabled and financially secure enjoys privileges that someone who is disabled and financially insecure does not. This is not to create hierarchies of oppression, but rather to identify for oneself and in society the ways that humans encounter one another and exert power in both interpersonal and systemic ways. Kimberlé W. Crenshaw, *On Intersectionality: Essential Writings* (New York: The New Press, 2017).

4   Here's a starting place. These anthologies include essays from a wide variety of fat, non-white, queer, trans, and disabled writers: Cat Pausé and Sonya Renee Taylor, eds., *The Routledge International Handbook of Fat Studies* (London: Routledge, 2021); Angie Manfredi, ed., *The (Other) F Word: A Celebration of the Fat and Fierce* (New York: Amulet Books, 2019); Bruce Owen Grimm, Miguel M. Morales, and Tiff Joshua TJ Ferentini, eds., *Fat and Queer: An Anthology of Queer and Trans Bodies and Lives* (London: Jessica Kingsley Publishers, 2021); Esther Rothblum and Sondra Solovay, eds., *The Fat Studies Reader* (New York: New York University Press, 2009).

5   Though, as we'll see, anti-fat bias in the United States has much older roots, mostly stemming from white supremacist encounters with non-white peoples, first through slavery and then through early nineteenth-

century xenophobia around immigration. The definitive book on this history is Sabrina Strings, *Fearing the Black Body: The Racial Origins of Fat Phobia* (New York: New York University Press, 2019).

6   Strings, *Fearing the Black Body*, 187–212; Harriet Brown, *Body of Truth: How Science, History, and Culture Drive our Obsession with Weight—and What We Can Do About It* (Boston: Da Capo Press, 2015), 1–32. For a quick overview—even though the article contains anti-fat bias—see Keith Devlin, "Top 10 Reasons Why the BMI is Bogus," *National Public Radio: Weekend Edition Saturday* (July 9, 2009), https://www.npr.org/templates/story/story.php?storyId=106268439.

7   Kindergartners are already socialized to show an aversion to larger bodies. When presented with pictures of children who are thin, average, and fat, children of all genders were shown to rank larger bodies last and describe them in negative ways. K.A. Kraig and P.K. Keel, "Weight-Based Stigmatization in Children," *International Journal of Obesity* 25 (2001): 1661–66.

8   Rebecca Puhl, "Weight Stigma Study in the U.S. and 5 Other Nations Shows the Worldwide Problem of Such Prejudice," *The Washington Post* (June 12, 2021).

9   Michelle M. Lelwica, *The Religion of Thinness: Satisfying the Spiritual Hungers behind Women's Obsession with Food and Weight* (Carlsbad, CA: Gürze Books, 2010).

10 James S. Puterbaugh, "The Emperor's Tailors: The Failure of the Medical Weight Loss Paradigm and its Causal Role in the Obesity of America," *Diabetes, Obesity, and Metabolism* 11, no. 6 (May 2009), 557–70; Ragen Chastain, "Do 95% of Dieters Really Fail?," June 28, 2011, https://danceswithfat.org/2011/06/28/do-95-of-dieters-really-fail/.

11 The trope of the "headless fatty" or "faceless fatty" is widely known and discussed in fat studies. The term originated in an essay by Charlotte Cooper in 2007 and gained traction as a shorthand for the usual negative media portrayal of fat people. See Charlotte Cooper, "Headless Fatties," 2007, http://charlottecooper.net/fat/fat-writing/headless-fatties-01-07/. Studying this phenomenon for the *Journal of Health Communication*, a team of researchers reinforced Cooper's observation, finding that seventy-two percent of images from news articles about weight and weight loss depicted fat people in a "negative, stigmatizing manner," often showing "only their abdomens or lower bodies, and to be shown eating or drinking." See Chelsea A. Heuer, Kimberly J. McClure, and Rebecca M. Puhl, "Obesity Stigma in Online News: A Visual Content Analysis," *Journal of Health Communication* 16, no. 9 (October 2011): 976–87, doi:

10.1080/10810730.2011.561915. Rebecca Alexander is the founder of AllGo, an app for the plus-sized community to access public spaces safely and comfortably (canweallgo.com). As a means of contesting the "faceless fatty" trope, she also introduced royalty-free stock photography of fat people (with heads!) doing all sorts of everyday tasks.

Chapter 1: A Big Fat Child of God

1   I know that use of the word "American" is reductive in many ways. The term "American" here refers both to my own national origin in the United States but also the ideals that undergird this nation—ideals like American exceptionalism, industrialization and automation, colonization and manifest destiny, white supremacy, and others. As we'll see, these and other ideals of American "civilization" undergird anti-fat bias. "American" is shorthand for the US context that I know best as both my frame of reference and primary research interest, but it is not intended to be understood as one monolithic culture. As I hope will become clear, while adipose tissue (fat) is a universal human biological fact, opinions around "fatness" are culturally constructed. For this reason, messages around "fat" vary widely in each ethnicity, region, and community in this country. When I say "American," it's to capture the overarching cultural messages that stream through US institutions such as the medical diet industry, food marketing, government, and media. These messages trickle down and are received differently from culture to culture, but their pervasiveness creates an overarching anti-fat narrative that is uniquely and importantly "American." Anti-fat hatred is yet another colonizing force that America has offered to the world. Fat activists, particularly those from non-white and non-US communities, have rightfully critiqued how much of fat discourse focuses on the white American context. And this is, indeed, the context from which I am writing. Naming this, I hope to underscore the limitations of this work for those who live beyond this cultural context. I invite all readers to explore works of fat activists in non-white and/or non-US locations. There is a diverse global conversation happening about the ways in which fat has been misunderstood and mistreated for capitalistic gain. This book is but one happy drop in that bucket.

2   Brené Brown, *I Thought It Was Just Me (but It Isn't): Making the Journey from "What Will People Think?" to "I Am Enough"* (New York: Penguin Random House, 2007), 4.

3   The seventy-eight-billion-dollar statistic comes from 2019: Marketdata, LLC, "Press Release: The U.S. Weight Loss & Diet Control Market," March 2021, https://www.researchandmarkets.com/reports/5313560/the-u-s-weight-loss-and-diet-control-market?w=4&utm_source=BW&utm_

medium=PressRelease&utm_code=qm2gts.

4   I started down the "bariatric surgery as cure" road a few times. I
    found that there are tremendous concerns over whether such extreme
    medical weight-loss interventions are ethical. These surgeries have
    a high on-the-table mortality rate, cause a host of chronic medical
    issues and perpetual malnutrition, and more than half of patients
    regain much or all of their previous weight over time. Even if I lost
    a significant amount of weight, I could easily be in worse physical
    shape afterwards. See Sarah Trainer, Alexandra Brewis, and Amber
    Wutich, *Extreme Weight Loss: Life Before and After Bariatric Surgery*
    (New York: New York University Press, 2021), 108–11; Lindo Bacon,
    Health at Every Size: The Surprising Truth About Your Weight (Dallas:
    Benbella Books, Inc., 2010), 62–66; Brown, *Body of Truth*, 99–100.
    Roxane Gay's beautiful essay on her decision to get bariatric surgery
    should be noted here, as well, because it shows the ambiguity with
    which she approached such a new encounter with her body before
    and after surgery: Roxane Gay, "What Fullness Is: On Getting Weight
    Reduction Surgery," *Medium*, April 24, 2018, https://gay.medium.com/
    the-body-that-understands-what-fullness-is-f2e40c40cd75.

5   The Venus of Willendorf is one of the oldest pieces of art ever
    uncovered: a small statue carved out of stone that was left in the ground
    over 25,000 years ago. She is of superfat or infinifat proportions. Sabrina
    Strings offers a discussion of her alongside other "venus" images in art
    history in her chapter "Being Venus" in *Fearing the Black Body*, 15–41.

6   Twin studies of ob*sity show that weight (like the more naturally
    understood factor of height) is highly correlated across time for people
    who share the same or similar genetic code. In other words, our genes
    often have much more to do with our body size than the diet industry
    would like us to believe. Why is this? How we process and store food
    has much to do with our internal chemistry and metabolism, which
    are genetically predisposed. Even hunger cues and satiety rates (how
    much we eat) are genetically intertwined. But the diet and medicalized
    weight-loss industries still need you to believe that your own personal
    choices are to blame for your fat so they can sell you products. An early
    twin study focused on ob*sity was Albert J. Stunkard, Terryl T. Foch,
    and Zdenek Hrubec, "A Twin Study of Human Obesity," *Journal of the
    American Medical Association* 256, no. 1 (1986): 51–54. See also Sondra
    Solovay, *Tipping the Scales of Justice: Fighting Weight-Based Discrimination*
    (Amherst, NY: Prometheus Books, 2000), 189–209. And the article Traci
    Mann and A. Janet Tomiyama, "What Thin People Don't Get About
    Dieting," *Chicago Tribune*, January 1, 2018.

7   For those not familiar, "crip theory" is a field of critical studies at the intersections of disability, capitalism, and queer embodiment. See Robert McRuer, *Crip Theory: Cultural Signs of Queerness and Disability* (New York: New York University Press, 2006); Rachel Hanebutt and Carlyn Mueller, "Disability Studies, Crip Theory, and Education," *Oxford Research Encyclopedia of Education*, February 23, 2021, https://doi.org/10.1093/acrefore/9780190264093.013.1392.

8   Michael Hobbes, "Everything You Know about Obesity is Wrong," *Huffington Post*, September 19, 2018, https://highline.huffingtonpost.com/articles/en/everything-you-know-about-obesity-is-wrong/.

9   Elena Levy-Navarro offers that "fat often functions as a master term that works in conjunction with other definitional nexuses, including those of race, sex, gender, and class . . . neither the category of fat nor the cultural phenomenon of fatphobia should be considered of lesser importance to other definitional terms and oppressions. Indeed, the extent to which the terms often work in concert should make us all more committed to considering their complex historical interdependence." Elena Levy-Navarro, ed., *Historicizing Fat in Anglo-American Culture* (Columbus: The Ohio State University Press, 2010), 3.

Chapter 2: The "F" Word

1   The currently average height of American women is five feet and four inches. Janet Morgan, "What Is the Average Height for Women," *Health Essentials*, April 21, 2021, https://health.clevelandclinic.org/what-is-the-average-height-for-women/.

2   Aubrey Gordon writing as Your Fat Friend, "Please, Just Call Me Fat," *Medium*, August 28, 2018, https://humanparts.medium.com/whos-hurt-by-being-called-fat-551930bc6989.

3   Thomas Baldwin, "Obesity and Public Health," presentation to the World Health Organization, November 2010, http://www.who.int/global_health_histories/seminars/presentation46a.pdf.

4   Kathleen LeBesco, "Fat Panic and the New Morality," in *Against Health: How Health Became the New Morality*, ed. Jonathan M. Metzl and Anna Kirkland (New York: New York University Press, 2010), 72–82; Aubrey Gordon, *What We Don't Talk About When We Talk About Fat* (Boston, MA: Beacon Press, 2020), 30–55; Paul Campos, Abigail Saguy, Paul Ernsberger, Eric Oliver, and Glenn Gaesser, "The Epidemiology of Overweight and Obesity: Public Health Crisis or Moral Panic?" *International Journal of Epidemiology* 35 (2006): 55–60.

5   Kathleen LeBesco, *Revolting Bodies: The Struggle to Redefine Fat Identity* (Amherst: University of Massachusetts Press, 2004), 29–39.

6   Cooper, *Fat Activism*, 51–95.

7   Strings, *Fearing the Black Body*.

8   Victoria Petersen, "Breaking Down the 'Wellness-Industrial Complex,' an Episode at a Time," *New York Times*, September 9, 2021, https://www.nytimes.com/2021/09/09/dining/wellness-industrial-complex-maintenance-phase.html. If you like *Maintenance Phase*, I suggest also listening to *Unsolicited: Fatties Talk Back*, a podcast co-hosted by five non-white and/or queer fat activists: Marquisele Mercedes, Da'Shaun Harrison, Caleb Luna, Bryan Guffey, and Jordan Underwood.

9   For a powerful discussion of anti-fatness, capitalism, and racialized violence, see Da'Shaun L. Harrison, *Belly of the Beast: The Politics of Anti-Fatness as Anti-Blackness* (Berkeley: North Atlantic Books, 2021).

10 Cooper self-describes as an oral history worker and is one of the founders of fat studies. See her website for information about her own research and her archiving efforts: http://charlottecooper.net. See also her personal blog, http://obesitytimebomb.blogspot.com/2015/12/archiving-fat-activism.html.

11 Laura Pratt, "The (Fat) Body and the Archive: Toward the Creation of a Fat Community Archive," *Fat Studies* 7, no. 2 (2018), https://doi.org/10.1080/21604851.2017.1374128.

12 Cat Pausé and Sonya Renee Taylor, "Fattening Up Scholarship," in Pausé and Taylor, *The Routledge International Handbook of Fat Studies,* 1–18.

13 Although, as ob*sity research continues to grow in its understanding of how weight stigma, rather than fat itself, negatively effects health outcomes, fat studies and some ob*sity studies may become aligned in their efforts to reduce societal harm to fat people. Still, ob*sity studies have to date functioned with the goal of ending ob*sity, and thus fat existence, which is antithetical to fat studies.

14 See the journal's homepage at https://www.tandfonline.com/toc/ufts20/current.

15 Fat shaming is a frequent phenomenon that has been shown to have negative health effects on fat people. If people believe they can shame someone into losing weight, they are extremely misguided. See A. Janet Tomiyama and Traci Mann, "If Shaming Reduced Obesity, There Would be No Fat People," *Hastings Center Report* (May 6, 2013).

16 Ash Nischuk's work can be found at thefatlip.com or @fatlip.ash on Instagram. Her taxonomy of fatness can be found in Aubrey Gordon, *What We Don't Talk About When We Talk About Fat*, 9–10.

17 The BMI is a problematic indicator of individual health. It is an overly simplified equation that was never meant to be used as a marker of health but rather to study the mathematical evolution of white European male sizes over time. Yet the BMI has been used as a standard in medical diagnosis, insurance coverage, and ob*sity treatments since the 1940s. The misclassification and stigmatization of patients on the basis of the BMI can lead to doctors unwilling to treat any ailments other than a person's size, a weight stigma that itself endangers fat people's lives. We will get into this more in future chapters, but some examples of ob*sity researchers themselves decrying the use of the BMI include: Richard V. Burkhauser and John Cawley, "Beyond BMI: The Value of More Accurate Measures of Fatness and Obesity in Social Science Research," *Journal of Health Economics* 27, no. 2 (March 2008): 519–29; R. M. Puhl and K. D. Brownell, "Psychosocial Origins of Obesity Stigma: Toward Changing a Powerful and Pervasive Bias," *Obesity Reviews* 4 (November 5, 2003), https://doi-org.ezproxy.bu.edu/10.1046/j.1467-789X.2003.00122.x.

18 Annette Richmond, "Ash of *The Fat Lip* Podcast Wants You to Know that Sizes above 32 Exist," *Ravishly*, February 26, 2018, https://www.ravishly.com/ash-fat-lip-podcast.

19 See Gordon, *What We Don't Talk About When We Talk About Fat*, 9–10.

Chapter 3: Dangerous but Liberative Unlearning

1 LeBesco, *Revolting Bodies*, 111–24.

2 Evelyn Higginbotham, *Righteous Discontent: The Women's Movement in the Black Baptist Church, 1880–1920* (Cambridge, MA: Harvard University Press, 1993).

3 Leah Donnella, "Where Does the 'Pull Up Your Pants' School of Black Politics Come From?" *Code Switch*, October 22, 2015, https://www.npr.org/sections/codeswitch/2015/10/22/450821244/where-does-the-pull-up-your-pants-school-of-black-politics-come-from.

4 Hobbes, "Everything You Know about Obesity is Wrong"; Campos, Saguy, Ernsberger, Oliver, and Gaesser, "The Epidemiology of Overweight and Obesity," 55.

5 J. Eric Oliver, *Fat Politics: The Real Story Behind America's Obesity Epidemic* (New York: Oxford University Press, 2006); Puterbaugh, "The Emperor's Tailors"; Brown, *Body of Truth*, 1–31.

6   Tessa E. S. Charlesworth and Mahzarin R. Banaji, "Patterns of Implicit and Explicit Attitudes: I. Long-Term Change and Stability From 2007 to 2016," *Psychological Science* 30, no. 2 (January 2019): 174–92, https://doi.org/10.1177%2F0956797618813087.

7   Ob*sity research often focuses its lens on non-white populations, particularly urban Black and Latinx communities, typically finding higher instances of ob*sity therein. However, too often these same studies fail to interrogate the link between racism and health disparity. What's more, these same ob*sity studies are often used to devalue racialized bodies further, assuming they are ignorant of how to "eat well" or claiming that these communities don't value "health" to the appropriate standard. This false narrative can become self-fulfilling prophesy as doctors render non-white bodies "social dead weight," and provide unequal healthcare for them. Author Sabrina Strings points to this racialized anti-fatness as a potential factor in the wide discrepancy in Covid-19 death rates between white and non-white populations. See Sabrina Strings, "It's Not Obesity, It's Slavery," *The New York Times*, May 25, 2020, https://www.nytimes.com/2020/05/25/opinion/coronavirus-race-obesity.html; Sabrina Strings, "Obese Black Women as 'Social Dead Weight': Reinventing the 'Diseased Black Woman'," *Journal of Women in Culture and Society* 41, no. 1 (Autumn 2015): 107–30.

8   In a widely read journal article, ob*sity researcher Dr. Daniel Callahan suggests increased "social pressure on the overweight," including personal shaming by doctors, is needed in the name of public health. Given the seventy-eight-billion-dollar diet industry, constant barrage of anti-fat marketing and media, and cultural shame placed on fat people every day, this is a maddening and worrisome suggestion. Daniel Callahan, "Obesity: Chasing an Elusive Epidemic," *Hastings Center Report* 43, no. 1 (February 2013): 34–40. Also, fat shaming has been shown to lead to increased weight gain, not loss. See Rebecca M. Puhl and Chelsea A. Heuer, "The Stigma of Obesity: A Review and Update," *Obesity: A Research Journal* (September 6, 2012), https://doi-org.ezproxy.bu.edu/10.1038/oby.2008.636.

9   Michelle M. Mello, David M. Studdert, and Troyen A. Brennan, "Obesity—The New Frontier of Public Health Law," *The New England Journal of Medicine* (June 15, 2006), https://doi.org/10.1056/nejmhpr060227.

10   Hobbes, "Everything You Know about Obesity is Wrong."

11   In 2019, Washington state became the first state in the United States to name "ob*sity" as a protected class, like gender and disability.

12 This thread was found on the American social media platform Quora, where people can ask and answer questions online. Similar questions were easily found by perfunctory searches on Twitter, Facebook, and Reddit.

13 Sonya Renee Taylor, *The Body is Not an Apology: The Power of Radical Self-Love* (Oakland, CA: Berrett-Koehler Publishers, 2018).

The Cookout

1   It may seem unusual that an eight-year-old would be placed on a commercial diet, but it is quite commonplace. Weight Watchers, or "WW" as they've rebranded themselves, recently launched "Kurbo," a weight-loss module made specially to target kids aged eight through seventeen. Girls as young as three to six report being dissatisfied with their body size and would prefer thinner bodies. See Sharon Hayes, "Am I Too Fat to Be a Princess: Examining the Effects of Popular Culture on Preschoolers' Body Image," PhD diss. (Orlando: University of Central Florida, 2008), https://stars.library.ucf.edu/cgi/viewcontent.cgi?article=4747&context=etd.

Section Two: Anti-Fat Bias, Its Origins, and Its Consequences

1   Cat Pausé, as quoted in "Everything You Know about Obesity is Wrong" by Michael Hobbes, *Huffington Post* (September 19, 2018). https://highline.huffingtonpost.com/articles/en/everything-you-know-about-obesity-is-wrong/.

Chapter 4: The Prevalence of Anti-Fat Bias

1   Sinead Gill, "Too Fat for NZ: Mum Can't Lose Weight Fast Enough for Immigration Officials," *Stuff*, June 26, 2021, https://www.stuff.co.nz/national/health/300341891/too-fat-for-nz-mum-cant-lose-weight-fast-enough-for-immigration-officials.

2   Nadeem Badshah, "Two Teenagers Placed in Foster Care after Weight Loss Plan Fails," *The Guardian*, March 11, 2021, https://www.theguardian.com/society/2021/mar/10/two-teenagers-placed-in-foster-care-after-weight-loss-plan-fails.

3   Ibid. Also, legal scholar Sondra Solovay discusses the regular occurrence of courts deeming fatness in children "child abuse" in her book *Tipping the Scales of Justice*, 13–24, 64–77.

4   Da'Shaun Harrison has been a primary voice criticizing the links between anti-fatness and police brutality in Black communities. Harrison, *Belly of the Beast*. They held a discussion with fat activist

Virgie Tovar that touches on this subject on Tovar's website and podcast *Rebel Eaters Club*: https://www.rebeleatersclub.com/episodes/dashaunharrison.

5   Michael R. Sisak, "Medical Examiner: Chokehold Triggered Eric Garner's Death," *AP News*, May 15, 2019, https://apnews.com/article/1903161fb60848a7851e68b25167f73b.

6   Alissa Scheller and Jan Diehm, "The Chokehold Is Banned by NYPD, but Complaints About Its Use Persist," *Huffpost,* December 5, 2014, https://www.huffpost.com/entry/nyc-police-chokeholds_n_6272000.

7   Rebecca Kukla, "Eric Garner and the Value of Black Obese Bodies," *Huffpost*, December 16, 2014, https://www.huffpost.com/entry/eric-garner-and-the-value-of-black-obese-bodies_b_6324568.

8   LeBesco, *Revolting Bodies*, 54–64 and 84–97.

9   Jane Lytvynenko, "The White Extremist Group Patriot Front Is Preparing for a World After Donald Trump," *BuzzFeed News*, October 27, 2020, https://www.buzzfeednews.com/article/janelytvynenko/patriot-front-preparing-after-trump.

10 Judith Hamera, "Weighty Anti-Feminism, Weighty Contradictions: Anti-Fat Coverage and Invective in US Right-Wing Populist Outlets," *Women's Studies* 48, no. 2 (2019): 146–66, https://doi.org/10.1080/00497878.2019.1580523.

11 Ann Coulter (@AnnCoulter), "Without fat girls, there would be no protests," Twitter, November 10, 2016, 12:28 p.m., https://twitter.com/AnnCoulter/status/796811901833478147.

12 Cat Pausé and Sandra Grey, "Throwing Our Weight Around: Fat Girls, Protest, and Civil Unrest," *M/C Journal* 21, no. 3, August 15, 2018, https://doi.org/10.5204/mcj.1424.

13 Its predecessor, the 21 Conference was established by an alt-right men's group in 2007 to get together and reclaim what it means to be a "real man." (Barf.) See Jonas Grinevičius, "$2,000 Tickets and All-Male Speakers: The 'Make Women Great Again' Convention is Causing Outrage on the Internet," *Bored Panda* (2020), https://www.boredpanda.com/make-women-great-again-22-convention/.

14 Ibid.

15 Ibid., emphasis in original.

16 Ibid.

17 Da'Shaun Harrison, "Fat People Must Become a Priority to the Left," *Wear Your Voice Magazine* (May 1, 2019), https://www.wearyourvoicemag.com/fatphobia-leftist-organizing/. See also their book: Harrison, *Belly of the Beast*.

18 Aubrey Gordon (under the pseudonym "Your Fat Friend"), "#MarALard*ss and the Left's Fat Problem," *Medium*, February 18, 2019, https://medium.com/@thefatshadow/maralard-ss-and-the-lefts-fat-problem-4dc57c498252.

19 Ibid.

20 "Fat, Sweaty Southerner in a White Suit," *TVTropes* (last modified May 20th, 2021), https://tvtropes.org/pmwiki/article_history.php?article=Main.FatSweatySouthernerInAWhiteSuit.

21 Fat activist and author Marianne Kirby pointed to how a popular political cartoon depicted a fat Covid-19 anti-vaccinator: "sitting on the ball part of a ball and chain that's attached to the ankle of a [thinner] bald person (maybe old) clawing their way toward a herd immunity finish line . . . so here we are, once again used as a symbol of selfish willful ignorance causing other people—more virtuous people—to suffer. This is exhausting. This is so painful. I CONCUR that antivaxxers are literally harming everyone at this point. But using fatness in this way… it actively harms fat people. And maybe you think it's fine to sacrifice fat folks because of the point about antivaxxers but I think that's shitty and you can do better. Please do better." Marianne Kirby (@TheRotund), Twitter, May 5, 2021, 12:04 p.m., https://twitter.com/TheRotund/status/1389974266058362880.

22 Pausé and Grey, "Throwing Our Weight Around."

23 Oliver, *Fat Politics*, 143–58.

24 Many non-white leaders decry food inequities, too, but their advocacy and action are rooted within their communities, not from outside. This means there is a much better understanding of and appreciation for complexity and systematic needs being met. See Shakirah Simley, "A More Abundant Share: The Future of Food is Black," *Huffington Post*, February 4, 2017, https://www.huffpost.com/entry/future-of-food-is-black_b_5895f081e4b0c1284f263d69.

25 Marquisele Mercedes, "Public Health's Power-Neutral, Fatphobic Obsession with 'Food Deserts'," *Medium*, November 13, 2020, https://marquisele.medium.com/public-healths-power-neutral-fatphobic-obsession-with-food-deserts-a8d740dea81.

26 Dr. Fatima Cody Stanford is a prominent ob*sity studies researcher whose research is funded in part by pharmaceutical companies seeking to sell weight loss drugs, such as Novo Nordisk. So, while her efforts to de-stigmatize ob*sity may be a positive step, her collective impact on fat people's wellbeing is still suspect. See Marquisele Mercedes's criticism of the too-cozy relationship between ob*sity researchers and diet drugs, "Wegovy Isn't a 'Game Changer', But an Update," MarquiseleMercedes. com, June 23, 2021, https://www.marquiselemercedes.com/writing/ wegovy.

27 Arianna MacNeill, "Racism and Obesity Are Inextricably Linked, Says a Harvard Doctor—and Here is How She Thinks That Can Change," *Boston.com*, April 12, 2021, https://www.boston.com/news/racial-justice/2021/04/12/ racism-and-obesity-article-fatima-cody-stanford-daniel-aaron/.

28 Ibid.

29 A thorough discussion of this problematic piece is found in Paul Campos, *The Obesity Myth: Why America's Obsession with Weight is Hazardous to Your Health* (New York: Gotham Books, 2004), 57–69.

30 As quoted in Campos, *The Obesity Myth*, 66.

31 The way queer Black culture has been appropriated by mainstream popular culture (read: white folks) is well-documented, and points to the issues inherent as marginalized groups gain representation and influence. Similarly, fat activists decry the ways that "body positivity," once a rallying cry for queer fat activists in the 1970s through 1990s, has now become appropriated to sell beauty, fashion, and "health" products rather than actually change society to be more size inclusive. See Cooper, *Fat Activism*, 14–17 and 145–52.

32 Sydneysky G., "Unraveling the Fatphobia Behind the Criticisms of Lizzo," *Wear Your Voice Mag*, December 13, 2019, https://www.wearyourvoicemag.com/ unraveling-the-fatphobia-behind-the-criticisms-of-lizzo/.

33 Amy Erdman Farrell, *Fat Shame: Stigma and the Fat Body in American Culture* (New York: New York University Press, 2011), 82–116.

34 Ibid., 19.

35 Healthism is a form of systemic bias that equates a lack of health with personal moral failure. See a fuller discussion of healthism and "healthist" bias in chapter 10.

36 Reid J. Epstein, "Liberals Eat Here. Conservatives Eat There," *The Wall Street Journal*, May 2, 2014, https://www.wsj.com/articles/BL-WB-45147.

37 Alex Abad-Santos, "SoulCycle Instructors Are as Mad About Its Investor's Trump Fundraiser as Its Riders Are," *Vox*, August 9, 2019, https://www.vox.com/2019/8/9/20791646/soulcycle-trump-fundraiser-backlash.

38 Erdman Farrell, *Fat Shame*, 13–17.

39 Wellness culture has recently come under scrutiny for applying these same principles to the Covid-19 pandemic in the form of vaccine skepticism. According to an article by Sirin Kale for *The Guardian,* just twelve wellness influencers were found to be responsible for nearly sixty-five percent of anti-vaccine content on Twitter and Facebook. See Sirin Kale, "Chakras, Crystals and Conspiracy Theories: How the Wellness Industry Turned its Back on Covid Science," *The Guardian*, November 11, 2021, https://www.theguardian.com/world/2021/nov/11/injecting-poison-will-never-make-you-healthy-how-the-wellness-industry-turned-its-back-on-covid-science.

40 Ibid.

41 Katherine Speller, "The Whole Foods Founder is Wrong About Nutrition & Food Access," *Yahoo!Life*, September 25, 2020, https://www.yahoo.com/lifestyle/whole-foods-founder-wrong-nutrition-232055007.html.

42 John Keefe, "Can You Tell a 'Trump' Fridge From a 'Biden' Fridge?," *The New York Times*, October 27, 2020, https://www.nytimes.com/interactive/2020/10/27/upshot/biden-trump-poll-quiz.html.

43 While this is not an exact quote, Guy Fieri and other Food Network stars regularly employ diet culture commentary alongside their recipes and reviews. My husband just watched the latest *Diners, Drive-ins, and Dives* (season 42, episode 5, March 11, 2022), and found two casually fatphobic references therein. (I still love you, Guy Fieri. Even if your casual fatphobia is unbecoming of the Mayor of Flavortown.)

Chapter 5: Women, Wasps, and Weight

1 Paul Starr, *The Social Transformation of American Medicine: The Rise of a Sovereign Profession and the Making of a Vast Industry* (New York: Basic Books, 2017), 32–35.

2 I've placed this word in quotes given that the growth of colonial "civilization" eradicated longstanding Indigenous civilizations that had existed long before colonists' arrival.

3   Strings, *Fearing the Black Body*, 122–46.

4   "Anglo-Saxon" refers to people of Northern European British ancestry, the ethnic lineage shared by most of the elite American colonists. Anglo-Saxon culture thereby dominated early American society and politics, and these cultural underpinnings have continued to influence American politics and society ever since.

5   I'm writing this on June 25, 2021, and the remains of 751 people have just been found in an unmarked grave at the site of a former Catholic school for Indigenous children in Canada. My God, the devastation Christianity has wrought supposedly in the name of the gospel, *kyrie eleison.* For an accounting of the Indigenous experience of colonial America see Roxanne Dunbar-Ortiz, *An Indigenous Peoples' History of the United States* (Boston: Beacon Press, 2015).

6   Strings, *Fearing the Black Body*, 6, 132–39.

7   Ibid., 70–71. The biological conception of race still pervades modern medicine, creating unhelpful diagnostic shorthand assumptions of patients on the basis of their ethnic origins. And yet the consensus among genetic and social scientists is that race is not a biological but a social construct. See Vivian Chou, "How Science and Genetics are Reshaping the Race Debate of the 21st Century," Science in the News Blog of Harvard University, April 17, 2017, https://sitn.hms.harvard.edu/flash/2017/science-genetics-reshaping-race-debate-21st-century/.

8   In her book *Superior: The Return of Race Science* (Boston: Beacon Press, 2019), Angela Saini traces the origins of racism in the medical industry, with an emphasis on how its legacy still enacts a caste-based system of health disparity for non-white Americans. Much medical research was (and still is) conducted on the premise that biological race—rather than societal disparities—is a causal factor of incongruent outcomes in public health.

9   Strings, *Fearing the Black Body*, 199.

10   As quoted in Adele Jackson-Gibson, "The Racist and Problematic History of the Body Mass Index," *Good Housekeeping*, February 23, 2021, https://www.goodhousekeeping.com/health/diet-nutrition/a35047103/bmi-racist-history/.

11   Strings, *Fearing the Black Body*, 199.

12   Ibid., 198.

13   Ibid., 198–200.

14 Jeremy Singer-Vine, "Beyond BMI: Why Doctors Won't Stop Using an Outdated Measure for Obesity," *Slate*, July 20, 2009, https://slate.com/technology/2009/07/why-are-doctors-still-measuring-obesity-with-the-body-mass-index.html.

15 Jayne Raisborough, "Turning Fat into Big Numbers," in *Fat Bodies, Health and the Media* (London: Palgrave Macmillan, 2016), 56–59.

16 Starr, *The Social Transformation of American Medicine*, 32–33.

17 Ibid., 34.

18 Ibid., 33.

19 Philip W. Ott, "John Wesley on Health as Wholeness," *Journal of Religion and Health* 30, no. 1 (Spring 1991): 43–57.

20 Ibid., 44–48.

21 Hillel Schwartz, *Never Satisfied: A Cultural History of Diets, Fantasies, and Fat* (New York: The Free Press, 1986), 23–46.

22 Oberlin College ended the Graham diet on its campus in 1841 after townspeople complained that its faculty and students appeared unsettlingly starved. Ibid., 44–46.

23 While I love a good Graham cracker, I think we can all agree they pale in comparison to the deliciousness of an orgasm.

24 Keeping ancestral bloodlines "pure" was a primary concern of elite whites in early America, since the concept of "race" recently had been established as an efficient way to pseudoscientifically categorize people into caste systems of advantage and disadvantage. See Isabel Wilkerson, *Caste: The Origins of Our Discontents* (New York: Random House), 2020.

25 Strings, *Fearing the Black Body*, 150–59.

26 Howard Markel and Alexandra Minna Stern, "The Foreignness of Germs: The Persistent Association of Immigrants and Disease in American Society," *The Millbank Quarterly* 80, no. 4 (December 2002): 757–88, https://doi.org/10.1111/1468-0009.00030.

27 Judith Walzer Leavitt, *Typhoid Mary: Captive to the Public's Health* (Boston: Beacon Press, 1996), 203.

28 Strings, *Fearing the Black Body*, 182.

29 Ibid., 173–82.

30 Kellogg's diet was likely inspired by the work of Sylvester Graham before him. Graham died the year before Kellogg was born, so the two men never met. However, both were influenced by the widespread nineteenth-century idea that masturbation could cause insanity. This and their shared Protestant piety for bodily control led them to believe that bland, vegetarian diets paired with lots of hydration could curb not only physical hunger but sexual appetites. See Matthew Wills, "The Strange Story Behind Your Breakfast Cereal," *JSTOR Daily,* February 26, 2019, https://daily.jstor.org/the-strange-backstory-behind-your-breakfast-cereal/. For more about nineteenth-century masturbation worries, see Vern L. Bullough, "Technology for the Prevention of 'Les Maladies Produites par la Masturbation'," *Technology and Culture* 28, no. 4 (October 1987): 828–32.

31 Strings, *Fearing the Black Body*, 175.

32 Wills, "The Strange Story Behind Your Breakfast Cereal."

33 Strings, *Fearing the Black Body*, 180–84.

34 Susan Bardo, "*Anorexia Nervosa:* Psychopathology as the Crystallization of Culture," in *Food and Culture: A Reader,* ed. Carole Counihan and Penny Van Esterik (New York: Routledge, 1997), 240–42.

35 Public health historian Ruth Clifford Engs has identified cycles of "clean living movements" that have occurred throughout the modern history of the United States. These sometimes decades-long movements arise from a conflation of public health concerns and moral panic about the state of society, often scapegoating a minoritized population as the source of disease or problematic living. The temperance (anti-alcohol) movement of the turn of the twentieth century is a well-known example, but others (for example, the "War on Drugs," "pro-life movement," and "AIDS crisis") have shown similar outcomes. Clean living movements arise when charismatic reformers (often with a sense of religious or moral urgency) target a particular behavior or lifestyle that they deem hazardous to the public good. When these reformers catch the attention of politicians or public health officials, campaigns of public policy and legislation are enacted to "clean up" society. Rather than helping, these efforts often further marginalize those people whose lifestyles were initially deemed dangerous. It is not a stretch to suggest that anti-fatness is currently reaching "clean living movement" proportions within the United States. Some fat activists are warning that legislative actions aimed at "cleaning up" fatness from society may soon arise, especially given the way ob*sity was scapegoated in the public health response to the Covid-19 pandemic. For more on historic clean living movements, see Ruth Clifford Engs, *Clean Living Movements: American Cycles of Health*

Reform (Westport, CT: Praeger Publishers, 2000). And for a look at fatness in the context of the Covid-19 pandemic, see Cat Pausé, George Parker, and Lesley Gray, "Resisting the Problematisation of Fatness in COVID-19: In Pursuit of Health Justice," *International Journal of Disaster Risk Reduction* 54 (February 15, 2021), https://doi.org/10.1016/j.ijdrr.2020.102021.

36 "Eugenics" is described thusly by Alexandra Stern: "[Eugenics] applied emerging theories of biology and genetics to human breeding. White elites with strong biases about who was 'fit' and 'unfit' embraced eugenics, believing American society would be improved by increased breeding of Anglo Saxons and Nordics, whom they assumed had high IQs. Anyone who did not fit this mold of racial perfection, which included most immigrants, Blacks, Indigenous people, poor whites and people with disabilities, became targets of eugenics programs. By 1913, many states had or were on their way to having eugenic sterilization laws . . . State-sanctioned sterilizations reached their peak in the 1930s and 1940s but continued and, in some states, rose during the 1950s and 1960s." Alexandra Stern, "Forced Sterilization Policies in the US Targeted Minorities and Those with Disabilities—And Lasted into the 21st Century," *IHPI News*, September 23, 2020, https://ihpi.umich.edu/news/forced-sterilization-policies-us-targeted-minorities-and-those-disabilities-and-lasted-21st.

37 Strings, *Fearing the Black Body*, 180–84.

38 As quoted in ibid., 144–45.

39 Schwartz, *Never Satisfied*, 91.

40 Ibid., 82–84.

41 Ibid., 160–61.

42 Lulu Hunt Peters, *Diet and Health: With Key to the Calories* (Chicago: The Reilly and Lee Co., 1918), 115–27.

43 Ibid., 84.

44 Ibid., 78–79.

45 The bodies of Hollywood actresses have always been scrutinized and critiqued with regard to their size. An article from the March 1931 issue of *Photoplay* magazine entitled "Who Has the Best Figure in Hollywood?" included a chart of the age, height, weight, bust, waist, hips, gloves, and shoe measurements of twenty-one starlets (all of them thin). See Anne Helen Petersen, "Judging the 'Best Figure in Hollywood,' 1931," *Slate,*

April 17, 2013, https://slate.com/human-interest/2013/04/best-figure-1931-photoplay-magazine-article-judges-starlet-measurements.html.

46 For a history of Depression-era food and its lasting legacy on how Americans eat still today, see Jane Ziegelman and Andrew Coe, *A Square Meal: A Culinary History of the Great Depression* (New York: Harper, 2016).

47 Amy Erdman Farrell notes how political cartoons have often included fatness as a visual cue for any number of problematic characteristics. See Farrell, *Fat Shame, 25–59.*

48 Schwartz, *Never Satisfied*, 141.

49 Ibid., 141.

50 Ibid., 142.

51 Bardo, "*Anorexia Nervosa:* Psychopathology as the Crystallization of Culture," 240.

52 Naomi Wolf's feminist classic *The Beauty Myth: How Images of Beauty Are Used Against Women* is an important book for anyone considering how capitalism and patriarchy align against women's power. However, a more recent work of hers included egregious research issues, and Wolf's wildly conspiratorial views on the Covid-19 pandemic and other topics got her banned from Twitter. I still feel that her work in *The Beauty Myth* is valuable, but I would be remiss if I did not complicate her herein as an author whose present-day scholarship is suspect. See Liza Featherstone, "The Madness of Naomi Wolf," *The New Republic*, June 10, 2021, https://newrepublic.com/article/162702/naomi-wolf-madness-feminist-icon-antivaxxer.

53 Naomi Wolf, *The Beauty Myth: How Images of Beauty Are Used Against Women* (New York: Harper Perennial, 2002), 61–66.

54 Jayne Raisborough, *Fat Bodies, Health and the Media* (London: Palgrave Macmillan, 2016), 17.

55 Wolf, *The Beauty Myth*, 65.

56 Nicolas Rasmussen points to the prevalence of psychology's effect on 1950s diet culture, which made the new, small group form of weight-loss intervention (like Weight Watchers) akin to other group therapy sessions that had been happening for some time. See Nicolas Rasmussen, *Fat in the Fifties: America's First Obesity Crisis* (Baltimore: Johns Hopkins University Press, 2019), 23–47.

57 Or what Susan Bardo calls "mammary madness," a beauty ideal glamorizing the large-breasted (but otherwise thin) woman that dominated popular American culture from the 1950s through early 1970s, until the British model Twiggy and 1980s workout culture arose. Bardo, "*Anorexia Nervosa:* Psychopathology as the Crystallization of Culture," 240–41.

58 Wolf, *The Beauty Myth*, 187.

59 Randall Balmer, "The Real Origins of the Religious Right," *Politico Magazine*, May 27, 2014, https://www.politico.com/magazine/story/2014/05/religious-right-real-origins-107133/.

60 Ibid.

61 Ibid.

62 LeBesco, *Revolting Bodies*, 29–39.

63 R. Marie Griffith, *Born Again Bodies: Flesh and Spirit in American Christianity* (Berkeley: University of California Press, 2004), 160–205. (But really, just read this whole book.)

64 Ibid., 4.

65 Strings, *Fearing the Black Body*, 194.

66 Schwartz, *Never Satisfied*, 332.

67 Judy Freespirit and Aldebaran, *Fat Liberation Manifesto* (Los Angeles: The Fat Underground/Largesse Fat Liberation Archives, 1973). Also found in Lisa Schoenfielder and Barb Wieser, eds., *Shadow on a Tightrope: Writings by Women on Fat Oppression* (San Francisco, CA: Aunt Lute Books, 1983), 52–53.

68 Farrell, *Fat Shame*, 143.

69 Wolf, *The Beauty Myth*, 187.

Chapter 6: The Polarizing Figure of the Unrepentant Fat Woman

1   Lelwica, *The Religion of Thinness*, 39.

2   "Dick Clark's Rockin' Eve" broadcasts the annual "ball drop" in New York's Times Square that marks for many Americans the start of the new year. For the past three years (2020–2022), the entire broadcast has been sponsored by Planet Fitness, a gym, which hands out its purple noisemakers and signs to the gathered crowd and peppers its

commercials throughout the broadcast. Among other commercials was one from Hill's Science Diet, a pet food chain, warning of the dangers of pet ob*sity. Nothing says "Happy New Year" like fat shaming Fido. But this underscores the fact that diet culture's New Year's push is extremely enculturated in America. Next year, notice how quickly Food Network pivots from decadent Christmas recipes in December to low-calorie New Years' resolution recipes in January.

3   LeBesco, *Revolting Bodies*, 54.

4   She coined the term on her blog: Lesley Kinzel, "Embracing the Morbid," *Two Whole Cakes Blog*, November 6, 2008, http://blog. twowholecakes.com/2008/11/embracing-the-morbid/. She uses the term further in her book Lesley Kinzel, *Two Whole Cakes: How to Stop Dieting and Learn to Love Your Body* (New York: The Feminist Press, 2012), 4, 63.

5   Campos, Saguy, Ernsberger, Oliver, and Gaesser, "The Epidemiology of Overweight and Obesity," 55–60.

6   LeBesco, *Revolting Bodies*, 56.

7   Ibid., 54–55.

8   Cooper, *Fat Activism*, 154–58. An expressed goal of the recent publication edited by Pausé and Taylor, *The Routledge International Handbook of Fat Studies,* was to bring a more diverse array of fat activist voices to the center of the conversation, particularly non-American, non-white voices. Fat white US women's voices (like mine) have been centered for the past twenty years. We overtook the narrative from the fat lesbians and trans women, often people of color, who were the revolutionary foremothers of the fat activism movement as early as the 1950s. An anthology capturing some of their voices is Schoenfielder and Wieser, *Shadow on a Tightrope*. Charlotte Cooper's *Fat Activism* captures the history of the fat activist movement from its origins to today.

9   This is not to say that non-white cultures equally embrace fatness. Anti-fat bias exists beyond American colonial reach, though it has certainly been globally exacerbated by the export of US beauty culture and media. Still, overall, fatness is understood to be less abject in collectivist cultures than in individualist ones. See LeBesco, *Revolting Bodies*, 56; Cindi SturtzSreetharan, Alexandra Brewis, Jessica Hardin, Sarah Trainer, and Amber Wutich, *Fat in Four Cultures: A Global Ethnography of Weight* (Toronto: University of Toronto Press, 2021).

10 Andrea Elizabeth Shaw, *The Embodiment of Disobedience: Fat Black Women's Unruly Political Bodies* (Lanham, MD: Lexington Books, 2006), 10.

11 Shaw's entire book is a gem, focusing on how society, through media and the entertainment industry, makes a "spectacle" of fat, Black women's bodies. Shaw, *The Embodiment of Disobedience*. Of similar interest is the excellent essay by Hunter Ashleigh Shackelford, "When You Are Already Dead: Black Fat Being as Afrofuturism," in Pausé and Taylor, *Routledge International Handbook of Fat Studies*, 253–57.

12 Joy Cox, "Truth Hurts: Lizzo, Black Women & Weight Stigma," *Center for Discovery Eating Disorder Treatment Website* (2019), https://centerfordiscovery.com/blog/truth-hurts-lizzo-black-women-weight-stigma/.

13 Shaw, *The Embodiment of Disobedience*, 99–126.

14 Ibid., 6–10.

15 Ibid.

16 See Stephanie Yeboah, *Fattily Ever After: A Black Fat Girl's Guide to Living Life Unapologetically* (London: Hardie Grant, 2020); Harrison, *Belly of the Beast*; Cooper, *Fat Activism*, 180–84; Virgie Tovar, *You Have the Right to Remain Fat* (New York: Feminist Press, 2018), 72.

17 LeBesco, *Revolting Bodies*, 47.

18 Cooper, *Fat Activism*, 12–16.

19 And dolls! Ruby, a size 16–18 version of Mattel's iconic waif the Barbie doll, was used in The Body Shop's 1998 ad campaign. The Body Shop was subsequently sued by Mattel for "denigrating" the image of Barbie.

20 Amena Azeez, "Being Fat in a Thin World: The Politics of Fashion," in Pausé and Taylor, *Routledge International Handbook of Fat Studies*, 117–19.

21 Tovar, *You Have the Right to Remain Fat*, 93.

22 Cooper, *Fat Activism*, 17.

Chapter 7: The Way We Understand "Fat" Is Cultural

1 Puterbaugh, "The Emperor's Tailors."

2 Tomiyama and Mann, "If Shaming Reduced Obesity, There Would Be No More Fat People."

3 The 1992 classic "Free Your Mind" from En Vogue's *Funky Divas* album was an R&B/rock/pop crossover call to examine one's own prejudices in

light of untrue stereotypes. For an all-Black female group to have a hit song decrying racism and misogyny was significant, even if some of the lyrics (like the ones inviting "colorblindness") have not aged well in the light of identity-first language and politics.

4   Brown, *Body of Truth*, xxvii.

5   Solovay, *Tipping the Scales of Justice*, 27.

6   Puterbaugh, "The Emperor's Tailors"; Chastain, "Do 95% of Dieters Really Fail?".

7   Kelly Crowe, "Obesity Research Confirms Long-Term Weight Loss Almost Impossible," *CBC News*, June 4, 2014, https://www.cbc.ca/news/health/obesity-research-confirms-long-term-weight-loss-almost-impossible-1.2663585.

8   For example, take the study by J. L. Kaaschnewski, J. Boan, J. Esposito, N. E. Sherwood, E. B. Lehman, D. K. Kephart, and C. N. Sciamanna, "Long-term Weight Loss Maintenance in the United States," *International Journal of Obesity* 34 (2010), 1664–54. They happily concluded, after finding that at least one-in-six people surveyed had sustained long-term weight-loss, "US adults may be more successful at sustaining weight loss than previously thought." The problem is their definition of "long-term" was only one year.

9   Traci Mann, *Secrets from the Eating Lab: The Science of Weight Loss, the Myth of Willpower, and Why You Should Never Diet Again* (New York: Harper Wave, 2017), 3.

10 These terms "yo-yo dieting" and "weight cycling" are attributed to ob*sity researcher Kelly D. Brownell of Duke University. An article about his work and the metabolic dangers of weight cycling can be found here: Gretchen Voss, "When You Lose Weight—and Gain It All Back," *NBC News*, June 6, 2010, https://www.nbcnews.com/health/health-news/when-you-lose-weight-gain-it-all-back-flna1c9446931.

11 Diane M. Quinn, Rebecca M. Puhl, and Mora A. Reinka, "Trying Again (and Again): Weight Cycling and Depressive Symptoms in U.S. Adults," *PLoS One* 15, no. 9 (September 11, 2020), https://doi.org/10.1371/journal.pone.0239004.

12 Traci Mann points to the fact that hundreds of studies have shown that dieters lose between five and fifteen pounds on average during the first four to six months of a diet, but that they hardly ever keep that weight off long-term. From Mann, *Secrets From the Eating Lab*, 3.

13 Kevin D. Hall and Scott Kahan, "Maintenance of Lost Weight and Long-Term Management of Obesity," *Medical Clinics of North America* 102, no. 1 (January 2018): 183–97, https://doi.org/10.1016/j.mcna.2017.08.012

14 Mann, *Secrets From the Eating Lab*, 33–50.

15 Erin Fothergill, Juen Guo, Lilian Howard, Jennifer C. Kerns, Nicolas D. Knuth, Robert Brychta, Kong Y. Chen, Monica C. Skarulis, Mary Walter, Peter J. Walter, and Kevin D. Hall, "Persistent Metabolic Adaptation 6 Years After 'The Biggest Loser' Competition," *Obesity* 24, no. 8 (August 2016): 1612–19, https://doi.org/10.1002/oby.21538.

16 As quoted in Kathryn Doyle, "6 Years After *The Biggest Loser*, Metabolism is Slower and Weight is Back Up," *Scientific American*, May 11, 2016, https://www.scientificamerican.com/article/6-years-after-the-biggest-loser-metabolism-is-slower-and-weight-is-back-up/.

17 To read more about how diets don't work, a place to start is Mann, *Secrets From the Eating Lab*. However, please note that Mann's work still returns to anti-fatness and healthist concerns about body size, so her work should be approached cautiously.

18 Quinn, Puhl, and Reinka, "Trying Again."

19 Using words like "normal" to describe smaller weights is itself a practice based in weight stigma.

20 Gina Kolata, "Genes Take Charge, and Diets Fall by the Wayside," *The New York Times*, May 8, 2007, https://www.nytimes.com/2007/05/08/health/08fat.html.

21 Solomon K. Musani, Stephen Erickson, and David B. Allison, "Obesity—Still Highly Heritable After All These Years," *American Journal of Clinical Nutrition* 87, no. 2 (February 2008): 275–76, https://doi.org/10.1002/oby.2153810.1093/ajcn/87.2.275.

22 Solovay, *Tipping the Scales of Justice*, 38.

23 Ethan A.H. Sims, "Destiny Rides Again as Twins Overeat," *New England Journal of Medicine* 322, no. 21 (June 1990): 1522–24, https://doi.org/10.1056/NEJM199005243222109; Kolata, "Genes Take Charge, and Diets Fall by the Wayside."

24 Quinn, Puhl, and Reinka, "Trying Again"; Peter Rzehak, Christa Meisinger, Gabriele Woelke, Sabine Brasche, Gert Strube, and Joachim Heinrich, "Weight Change, Weight Cycling and Mortality in the ERFORT Male Cohort Study," *European Journal of Epidemiology* 22, no. 10 (2007):

665–73, https://doi.org/10.1007/s10654-007-9167-5; Voss, "When You Lose Weight—and Gain it All Back."

25 As quoted in Laura Fraser, "The Inner Corset: A Brief History of Fat in the United States," in Rothblum and Solovay, *The Fat Studies Reader*, 11–14. It's interesting to note the gendered language of the "fat man" and "thin woman," though. Perhaps Dr. Hutchinson was foreshadowing the attention that would mostly be paid to women's weights over the next hundred plus years.

26 Donna Ciliska, "Set Point: What Your Body is Trying to Tell You," *National Eating Disorder Information Centre*, available as a PDF download from https://nedic.ca/.

27 Brown, *Body of Truth*, xv–xxvii.

28 A few great histories of cultural fatness in the United States are Levy-Navarro, *Historicizing Fat in Anglo-American Culture*; Schwartz, *Never Satisfied*; Strings, *Fearing the Black Body*; Oliver, *Fat Politics*; Erdman Farrell, *Fat Shame*.

29 Former Surgeon General C. Everett Koop declared a public "War on Fat" in 1994, which he called a personal "crusade" after he lost twenty-five pounds. Koop cited statistics on the mortality rates and health care costs of ob*sity that since have been debunked as exaggerations by many scientists, including the *New England Journal of Medicine*. See LeBesco, *Revolting Bodies*, 29–39; Erdman Farrell, *Fat Shame*, 13–14; and an article from the time, Russ Loar, "Doctor's Orders: Ex-Surgeon General Koop Calls for War Against Obesity," *Los Angeles Times*, March 18, 1995, https://www.latimes.com/archives/la-xpm-1995-03-18-me-44239-story.html.

30 Many authors describe the unholy alliance of weight-loss marketing and the medical establishment. For a tremendous overview of it from a diet pharmaceutical standpoint, see Alicia Mundy, *Dispensing with the Truth: The Victims, the Drug Companies, and the Dramatic Story Behind the Battle Over Fen-Phen* (New York: St. Martin's Press, 2001).

31 Ibid., 41–42.

32 LeBesco, "Fat Panic and the New Morality," 72–75.

33 Brown, *Body of Truth*, 100–107. Make sure to check out Dr. Deb Burgard's excellent chart on page 106.

34 Oliver, *Fat Politics*, 5–8.

35 Campos, Saguy, Ernsberger, Oliver, and Gaesser, "The Epidemiology of Overweight and Obesity."

36 Oliver, *Fat Politics*, 1–2.

37 Raisborough, *Fat Bodies, Health and the Media*, 9–12, 51–76.

38 Erdman Farrell, *Fat Shame*, 9–10.

Chapter 8: An Unholy Trinity: The Diet, Beauty, and Medical Industries

1 Taylor, *The Body is Not an Apology*, 39.

2 Julie Guthman, *Weighing In: Obesity, Food Justice, and the Limits of Capitalism* (Berkeley: University of California Press, 2011), 163.

3 The 2022 annual report on the financial state of the weight-loss industry, compiled by Marketdata, LLC, was released in March 2022. Marketdata, LLC, "U.S. Weight Loss Market Shrinks 25% in 2020, but Rebounds in 2021," March 4, 2022, https://www.marketdataenterprises.com/u-s-weight-loss-market-shrinks-25-in-2020-but-rebounds-in-2021/.

4 Ibid.

5 Marketdata, LLC, "Press Release: The U.S. Weight Loss & Diet Control Market," March 2021, https://www.researchandmarkets.com/reports/5313560/the-u-s-weight-loss-and-diet-control-market.

6 Bee Wilson, "Why We Fell for Clean Eating," *The Guardian*, August 11, 2017, https://www.theguardian.com/lifeandstyle/2017/aug/11/why-we-fell-for-clean-eating.

7 Daniel Lefferts, "Diets for Mere Mortals: Health & Fitness Books 2018–2019," *Publishers Weekly*, November 2, 2018, https://www.publishersweekly.com/pw/by-topic/new-titles/adult-announcements/article/78494-diets-for-mere-mortals-health-and-fitness-books-2018-2019.html.

8 Caroline Dooner, *The F*ck It Diet: Eating Should be Easy* (New York: Harper Wave, 2019).

9 Ibid., 4–5.

10 Marie Galmiche, Pierre Déchelotte, Grégory Lambert, and Marie Pierre Tavolacci, "Prevalence of Eating Disorders Over the 2000–2018 Period: A Systematic Literature Review," *The American Journal of Clinical Nutrition*, 109, no. 5 (May 2019): 1402–13, https://doi.org/10.1093/ajcn/nqy342.

11 Wilson, "Why We Fell for Clean Eating." Please note the echoes of Dr. Kellogg's popular "clean eating" regimen of the early twentieth century discussed in chapter 5.

12 Eric Graber, "Eating Disorders Are on the Rise," *American Society for Nutrition*, February 22, 2021, https://nutrition.org/eating-disorders-are-on-the-rise/.

13 On December 8, 2021, the *New York Times* published an article by Roni Caryn Rabin entitled "The Coronavirus Attacks Fat Tissue, Scientists Find," with the lead line, "The research may help explain why people who are overweight and obese have been at higher risk of severe illness and death from Covid," https://www.nytimes.com/2021/12/08/health/covid-fat-obesity.html. However, this *New York Times* article (which spread over social media like the clickbait it was intended to be) was based on one single, not-yet-peer-reviewed-or-published study of eleven people's cell samples, only three of whom were living at the time, and seven of whom were over the age of sixty-five. See Virginia Sole-Smith's essay "Covid, Fat Cells, and Journalism's Personal Responsibility Problem," *Burnt Toast*, December 21, 2021, https://virginiasolesmith.substack.com/p/covid-fat-cells-and-journalisms-personal. Sole-Smith is quick to point out how anti-fat bias in both medicine and media have been hallmarks of this country's response to the coronavirus pandemic. If government officials can place personal blame on the virus' victims as particularly vulnerable, rather than admitting systemic governmental public health response failures, then the country can get "back to normal" and only risk those who "don't take care of themselves" and are thereby not considered worthy of care.

14 Monica Melton, "Weight Loss App Noom Quadruples Revenue Again, This Time to $237 Million," *Forbes*, January 14, 2020, https://www.forbes.com/sites/monicamelton/2020/01/14/weight-loss-app-noom-quadruples-revenue-again-this-time-to-237-million/?sh=226fe11660f2.

15 Ibid.

16 Amrita Khalid, "How Noom Won 2020, A Banner Year for Wellness and Weight-Loss Apps," *Inc.com*, May 18, 2021, https://www.inc.com/amrita-khalid/noom-saeju-jeong-weight-loss-app.html.

17 Tom Foster, "How Noom's Founders Shook Up a $250 Billion Industry with a Pandemic Hit That Took 10 Years to Build," *Inc. Magazine,* Winter 2021/2022, https://www.inc.com/magazine/202112/tom-foster/noom-weight-loss-behavior-app-saeju-jeong-artem-petakov.html.

18 It may not be a private company for long. Noom is said to be considering going public with an IPO valued at ten billion dollars. See ibid.

19 "Front Page," Noom.com.

20 Avi Dan, "The Weight Watchers Rebrand Points to the Risk of Chasing Trends," *Forbes*, April 11, 2019, https://www.forbes.com/sites/avidan/2019/04/11/the-weight-watchers-rebrand-points-to-the-risk-of-chasing-trends/.

21 Jess Walton, "Losing My Religion," in Manfredi, *The (Other) F Word*, 138–44.

22 Rebecca Scritchfield, "Weight Watchers is Targeting Teens with a New Free Program. That's a Problem: When We Send Kids the Message That a Number on the Scale is Most Important, They Suffer," *The Washington Post*, February 9, 2018; Brown, *Body of Truth*, 48–56.

23 Erdman Farrell, *Fat Shame*, 13–14.

24 Virginia Sole-Smith, "In Obesity Research, Fatphobia is Always the X Factor," *Scientific American*, March 6, 2021, https://www.scientificamerican.com/article/in-obesity-research-fatphobia-is-always-the-x-factor/.

25 Stella Medvedyuk, Ahmednur Ali, and Dennis Raphael, "Ideology, Obesity, and the Social Determinants of Health: A Critical Analysis of the Obesity and Health Relationship," *Critical Public Health* 28, no. 5 (2018): 573–85; Jane E. Brody, "Fat Bias Starts Early and Takes a Serious Toll," *The New York Times*, August 21, 2017, https://www.nytimes.com/2017/08/21/well/live/fat-bias-starts-early-and-takes-a-serious-toll.html.

26 Hobbes, "Everything You Know About Obesity is Wrong."

27 Puhl and Heuer, "The Stigma of Obesity." See also this article with a great amount of implicit weight stigma, but nonetheless interesting: Asia M. Friedman, Jennifer R. Hemler, Elisa Rossetti, Lynn P. Clemow, and Jeanne M. Ferrante, "Obese Women's Barriers to Mammography and Pap Smear: The Possible Role of Personality," *Obesity* 20, no. 8 (August 2012): 1611–17, https://dx.doi.org/10.1038%2Foby.2012.50.

28 As quoted in American Psychological Association, "Press Release: Fat Shaming in the Doctor's Office Can Be Mentally and Physically Harmful," August 3, 2017, https://www.apa.org/news/press/releases/2017/08/fat-shaming.

29 Medvedyuk, Ali, and Raphael, "Ideology, Obesity and the Social Determinants of Health."

30 Beth Sayan, *Science Under Siege: The Myth of Objectivity in Scientific Research* (Montréal: CBC Enterprises, 1988).

31 Natalie Boero, *Killer Fat: Media, Medicine, and Morals in the American "Obesity Epidemic"* (New Brunswick, NJ: Rutgers University Press, 2013); Raisborough, *Fat Bodies, Health and the Media.*

32 David P. Miller, Jr., John G. Spangler, Mara Z. Vitolins, Stephen W. Davis, Edward H. Ip, Gail S. Marion, and Sonia J. Crandall, "Are Medical Students Aware of Their Anti-obesity Bias?" *Academic Medicine* 88, no. 7 (July 2013): 978–82, https://doi.org/10.1097/ACM.0b013e318294f817. In this three-year longitudinal study, authors interviewed all third-year medical students going through the Wake Forest School of Medicine (n=310) and had them take the "Weight Implicit Association Test" to determine the extent to which they were biased by body size. Thirty-three percent were considered "strongly biased" against fat bodies, and an additional thirty-nine percent were seen to be implicitly biased (they would not name themselves as biased, but the results of their test showed bias). Sixty-seven percent of participants said they were unaware they held any anti-fat bias. And for the effects of anti-fat bias in medical industry, see Hobbes, "Everything You Know About Obesity is Wrong."

33 Katherine M. Flegal, Brian K. Kit, Heather Orpana, and Barry I. Graubard, "Association of All-Cause Mortality with Overweight and Obesity Using Standard Body Mass Index Categories: A Systematic Review and Meta-Analysis," *Journal of the American Medical Association* 309, no. 1 (January 2013): 71–82, https://doi.org/10.1001/jama.2012.113905; Mann, *Secrets from the Eating Lab,* 67–88.

34 Brown, *Body of Truth,* 29–31; Katherine M. Flegal and Kamyar Kalantar-Zadeh, "Perspective: Overweight, Mortality and Survival," *Obesity* 21, no. 9 (September 2013): 1744–45, https://doi.org/10.1002/oby.20588.

35 Brown, *Body of Truth,* 45–46.

36 Campos, Saguy, Ernsberger, Oliver, and Gaesser, "The Epidemiology of Overweight and Obesity."

37 This is a reference to the classic Hans Christian Andersen tale "The Emperor's New Clothes," in which an enterprising pair of crooks trick a haughty emperor into believing he has purchased magnificent, though invisible, clothing. Everyone goes along with the ruse, not wanting to enrage or embarrass the emperor, who parades through the town in his naked glory, thinking himself well-dressed. Only when a child points out the emperor's nakedness does the crowd admit that they, too, realized he was naked all along. It was just that no one wanted to be the first to say it. Puterbaugh is suggesting that ob*sity researchers similarly understand the fact that weight-loss interventions actually cause weight gain and

yet refuse to end the medical weight loss paradigm. Puterbaugh, "The Emperor's Tailors."

38 Ibid.

39 Ibid.

40 Project Implicit was founded by three researchers—Tony Greenwald, Mahzarin Banaji, and Brian Nosek—in 1998, and the tests can be found on the Project Implicit website: https://implicit.harvard.edu/implicit/selectatest.html.

41 Charlesworth and Banaji, "Patterns of Implicit and Explicit Attitudes."

42 A version of the IAT where the subject is asked to react to pictures of fatter faces vs. thinner faces. Charlesworth and Banaji, "Patterns of Implicit and Explicit Attitudes."

43 Gordon, *What We Don't Talk About When We Talk About Fat*, 23–25.

44 Ibid., 25.

45 Erdman Farrell, *Fat Shame*, 131–35.

46 Phil Edwards, "A Brief History of the Bizarre and Sadistic Presidential Fitness Test," *Vox*, April 24, 2015, https://www.vox.com/2015/4/24/8489501/presidential-fitness-test; Campos, *The Obesity Myth*, 185–98.

47 Kraig and Keel, "Weight-based Stigmatization in Children."

48 Brody, "Fat Bias Starts Early."

49 Ancel Keys, Josef Brozek, et al., *The Biology of Human Starvation,* vols. 1–2 (Minneapolis, MN: University of Minnesota Press, 1950).

50 Solovay, *Tipping the Scales of Justice*, 196.

51 Caroline Dooner offers a full description of the experiment and its implications in her book, *The F*ck It Diet*, 18–24. See also Solovay, *Tipping the Scales of Justice*, 196–200.

52 Dooner, *The F*ck It Diet*, 19.

53 Solovay, *Tipping the Scales of Justice*, 197.

54 Ibid., 197–98; Dooner, *The F*ck It Diet*, 20–21.

55 Dooner, *The F*ck It Diet*, 20.

56 Solovay, *Tipping the Scales of Justice*, 198.

57 Dooner, *The F*ck It Diet*, 22.

58 Solovay, *Tipping the Scales of Justice*, 198–99.

59 Dooner, *The F*ck It Diet*, 23.

60 Ibid.

61 Solovay, *Tipping the Scales of Justice*, 199.

62 Medvedyuk, Ali, and Raphael, "Ideology, Obesity, and the Social Determinants of Health."

63 A number of "mindful eating" and "intuitive eating" books have come out lately offering this same advice. However, most were written by non-fat nutritionists, doctors, and public health officials who take anti-fatness as a given and promote weight loss. Many of these books promise bodily "set points" within a "normal" medical range if their mindfulness practices are applied. This is still anti-fat diet culture at work! Trusting one's own internal cues of hunger and satiety is difficult for many fat people because of the ways our bodies have been regimented by restrictive dieting. "Eating normally" makes no physical sense to someone like me who grew up on fifteen different diet plans. "Mindfulness" eating is just another diet plan. For mindful eating to be weight neutral in its approach, it must focus not only on eating slowly to the point of fullness but also dismantling moralizing narratives around various foods, embracing the pleasure of eating purely for fun or comfort, and—importantly—ending the weight-loss mentality altogether. For mindful eating to be fat liberationist, it would need to address and then seek to change the structures of oppression and capitalism that cause only but the most privileged to have time, energy, and money enough to eat "mindfully" in the first place.

64 Please see the footnote above. It's difficult for me to recommend any books by nutritionists or doctors, given how much their work depends on anti-fatness. Still, here are a few that aren't perfect, but don't actively disgust me: Tansy Boggon, *Joyful Eating: How to Break Free of Diets and Make Peace with Your Body* (Lulu Publishing, 2021); Laura Thomas, *Just Eat It: How Intuitive Eating Can Help You Get Your Shit Together Around Food* (London: Bluebird, 2019); Joshua Wolrich, *Food Isn't Medicine* (London: Vermilion, 2021); Bacon, *Health at Every Size*.

Chapter 9: Big Fat Truths About Ob*sity

1 Norbert Stefan, Konstantinos Kantarzis, and Jürgen Machann, "Identification and Characterization of Metabolically Benign Obesity

in Humans," *Archives of Internal Medicine* 168, no. 15 (2008): 1609–16, https://doi.org/10.1001/archinte.168.15.1609; Ethan A.H. Sims, "Are There Persons Who Are Obese, But Metabolically Healthy?" *Metabolism* 50, no. 12 (January 2002): 1499–1504, https://doi.org/10.1053/meta.2001.27213.

2   Campos, *The Obesity Myth*.

3   Sirena Bergman, "Society Insists that Laziness Makes Us Fat—Now Science Proves This is Baseless Bigotry," *The Independent*, January 25, 2019, https://www.independent.co.uk/voices/fat-overweight-dna-study-thin-people-women-tess-holliday-donald-trump-a8746166.html.

4   Hobbes, "Everything You Know About Obesity Is Wrong."

5   Pat Lyons, "Prescription for Harm: Diet Industry Influence, Public Health Policy, and the 'Obesity Epidemic'," in Rothblum and Solovay, *The Fat Studies Reader*, 75–87.

6   Campos, *The Obesity Myth*, 119–30; Mann, *Secrets From the Eating Lab*, 51–88.

7   Brown, *Body of Truth*, 1–31; Traci Mann, *Secrets from the Eating Lab*, 3–67.

8   Doctor Tim Caulfield, who critiques the medical discourse around ob*sity and weight loss, describes it thusly, "You go to these meetings and you talk to researchers, you get a sense there is almost a political correctness around it, that we don't want this message [that sustained weight-loss isn't possible] to get out there." Quoted in Crowe, "Obesity Research." Caulfield's book *The Cure For Everything* further describes the misinformation campaigns of medical weight loss, diet industry, and fitness experts: Timothy Caulfield, *The Cure For Everything: Untangling Twisted Messages About Health, Fitness, and Happiness* (Boston: Beacon Press, 2012), 43–98. Please note that even critics of ob*sity research, like Caulfield, are not impervious to anti-fat bias and sizeism.

9   Harriet Brown, "The Weight of the Evidence," *Slate Magazine*, March 24, 2015, https://slate.com/technology/2015/03/diets-do-not-work-the-thin-evidence-that-losing-weight-makes-you-healthier.html.

10 Alice M. Arnold, Anne B. Newman, Mary Cushman, Jingzhong Ding, Stephen Kritchevsky, "Body Weight Dynamics and Their Associations with Physical Function and Mortality in Older Adults: The Cardiovascular Health Study," *The Journals of Gerontology: Series A* 65A, no. 1 (January 2010): 63–70, https://doi.org/10.1093/gerona/glp050; Rhee EJ, Cho JH, Kwon H, Park SE, Park CY, Oh KW, Park SW, and Lee WY, "Increased Risk of Diabetes Development in Individuals

with Weight Cycling Over 4 Years: The Kangbuk Samsung Health Study," *Diabetes Research in Clinical Practice* 139 (May 2018): 230–38, https://doi.org/10.1016/j.diabres.2018.03.018.

11 Brown, *Body of Truth*, 48–49.

12 Bacon, *Health at Every Size*, 46–50; Paul Ernsberger, "Foreword," in Campos, *The Obesity Myth*, x.

13 A. Janet Tomiyama, Britt Ahlstrom, and Traci Mann, "Long-term Effects of Dieting: Is Weight Loss Related to Health?" *Social and Personality Psychology Compass* 7, no. 12 (2013): 861–77; Traci Mann, A. Janet Tomiyama, Erika Westling, Ann-Marie Lew, Barbara Samuels, and Jason Chatman, "Medicare's Search for Effective Obesity Treatments: Diets Are Not the Answer," *American Psychologist* 62, no. 3 (April 2007): 220–33.

14 Puterbaugh, "The Emperor's Tailors."

15 Aubrey Gordon, writing as Your Fat Friend, "The Way We Talk About Our Bodies is Deeply Flawed," *Medium*, April 23, 2019, https://humanparts.medium.com/the-problem-with-how-we-talk-about-our-bodies-443fbc36875e.

16 Ibid.

17 Christy Harrison, "What Thin Privilege Really Means," May 7, 2019, https://christyharrison.com/blog/what-is-thin-privilege.

18 Kinzel, *Two Whole Cakes*, 8.

19 Krista Casazza, et al., "Weighing the Evidence of Common Beliefs in Obesity Research," *Critical Reviews in Food Science and Nutrition* 55, no. 14 (December 6, 2015): 2014–53.

20 Ibid.

21 Francesco Rubino, et al., "Joint International Consensus Statement for Ending Stigma of Obesity," *Nature Medicine* 26 (2020): 485–97, https://doi.org/10.1038/s41591-020-0803-x.

22 Ibid.

23 Ibid.

24 Campos, Saguy, Ernsberger, Oliver, and Gaesser, "The Epidemiology of Overweight and Obesity."

25 Ibid.

26 Jeanne Sager, "Most Americans Are Too Fat to Donate Their Bodies to Science," *Vice*, March 14, 2017, https://www.vice.com/en/article/vvjz3d/most-americans-are-too-fat-to-donate-their-bodies-to-science.

27 Mandy Oaklander, "Why You Probably Can't Donate a Kidney Even if You Want To," *Time*, November 14, 2014, https://time.com/3585545/kidney-donation-obesity/.

28 Sager, "Most Americans Are Too Fat to Donate Their Bodies to Science."

29 Janice A. Sabin, Maddalena Marini, and Brian A. Nosek, "Implicit and Explicit Anti-Fat Bias Among a Large Sample of Medical Doctors by BMI, Race/Ethinicity and Gender," *PLOS One*, November 7, 2012, https://doi.org/10.1371/journal.pone.0048448.

30 The show is based on Lindy West's memories as a fat woman. There is a difference, however, between Lindy West's size and actor Aidy Bryant's. Aidy is much smaller both in stature and in size. So, while Aidy is awesome in the role of Annie, it's interesting that even in *Shrill*, Hollywood downsizes visual fatness. How much more radical might the show have been to see someone superfat or larger on the screen in that role? As fat representation widens on the small and big screens, perhaps one day there will be room for the largest bodies. I hope so.

31 Marie Southard Ospina, "Shrill is the First Show to Accurately Portray Fat Women's Experiences," *Dazed*, December 27, 2019, https://www.dazeddigital.com/beauty/body/article/47297/1/shrill-tv-show-fat-plus-size-women-acceptance-self-worth-hulu-community.

32 Fat people are not the only ones with the experience of being dismissed by health care providers. One's perceived race can also play a role in the quality of care received. Nancy Krieger of Harvard's Chan School of Public Health has found premature death rates among African Americans living in states where Jim Crow laws were once prevalent. See Ericka Stallings, "The Article That Could Help Save Black Women's Lives," *O Magazine*, October 2018, https://www.oprah.com/health_wellness/the-article-that-could-help-save-black-womens-lives#ixzz5VRnkBHiz.; Nancy Krieger, Jaquelyn L. Jahn, Pamela D. Waterman, and Jarvis T. Chen, "Breast Cancer Estrogen Receptor Status According to Biological Generation: US Black and White Women Born 1915–1979," *American Journal of Epidemiology* 187, no. 5 (May 1, 2018): 960–70, https://doi.org/10.1093/aje/kwx312.

33 Angela S. Alberga, Iyoma Y. Edache, Mary Forhan, and Shelly Russell-Mayhew, "Weight Bias and Health Care Utilization: A Scoping Review," *Primary Health Care Research & Development* 20 (July 22, 2019), https://

doi.org/10.1017/S1463423619000227; N. K. Amy, A. Aalborg, P. Lyons, et al., "Barriers to Routine Gynecological Cancer Screening for White and African-American Obese Women," *International Journal of Obesity* 30 (January 1, 2006): 147–55, https://doi.org/10.1038/sj.ijo.0803105.

34 There is a term in the field of trauma studies for the experience of an institution knowingly reversing victim and offender: institutional betrayal. This concept was introduced by Jennifer J. Freyd and has since been explored by Freyd and Pamela Birrell in their book *Blind to Betrayal* (Hoboken, NJ: John Wiley & Sons, 2013), and in the article "Institutional Betrayal," *American Psychologist* 69, no. 6 (September 2014): 575–87, http://dx.doi.org/10.1037/a0037564. A particularly insidious form of institutional betrayal goes by the acronym "DARVO," which stands for "Defend, Attack, Reverse Victim and Offender." This is a three-step process by which the offending institution or individual not only denies culpability but reverses the narrative to attack the victim, placing blame on the victim in order to minimize the institution's own wrongdoing. Medicalized anti-fatness can be understood within the framework of DARVO and institutional betrayal given that diet culture's negative health effects are widely known in the medical field—yet doctors continue to blame fat people for their own ill-health.

35 Hobbes, "Everything You Know about Obesity Is Wrong."

36 Ragen Chastain, "Doctor's E-mails Expose Their Fatphobia," *Dances With Fat* (blog), January 17, 2020, https://danceswithfat.org/2020/01/17/doctors-e-mails-expose-their-fatphobia/.

37 Brown, *Body of Truth*, 9.

38 Just as a tip-of-the-iceberg starting place, see Hobbes, "Everything You Know about Obesity Is Wrong."

39 Lyons, "Prescription for Harm."

40 Mann, *Secrets from the Eating Lab*, 8–9.

41 See the discussions of Nutri-System and unregulated diet plans in Solovay, *Tipping the Scales of Justice*, 171–89.

42 Mann, *Secrets from the Eating Lab*, 9.

Chapter 10: The Question of "Health"

1   What is "health," even? I keep the quotations around this word because it is so ambiguous. Is one "healthy" if they "look healthy," don't have any physical ailments, or just feel good? Is one "healthy" when they live

longer than their peers? But what about the natural diseases of old age as the body atrophies? Harriet Brown discusses the thorniness of even defining "health" as a concept. See Brown, *Body of Truth*, 7–9.

2   Cooper, *Fat Activism*, 184–87.

3   See April Herndon, "Disparate but Disabled: Fat Embodiment and Disability Studies," *NWSA Journal* 14, no. 3 (Autumn 2002): 120–37; Gemma Gibson, "Health(ism) At Every Size: The Duties of the 'Good Fatty,'" *Fat Studies*, April 9, 2021, https://doi.org/10.1080/21604851.2021.1906526; LeBesco, *Revolting Bodies*, 111–24.

4   LeBesco, *Revolting Bodies*, 54–64.

5   Most fat haters aren't so articulate in their critique. They just say, "Moo—no one will ever love you, cow." Or much worse. What better way to dehumanize fat people than to make an animal comparison? Fat haters, when you come for me, please know that I prefer to be compared to manatees because sailors used to mistake them for mermaids. Think about that for a second. All these drawings of thin mermaids are historically wrong.

6   Campos, Saguy, Ernsberger, Oliver, and Gaesser, "The Epidemiology of Overweight and Obesity"; Campos, *The Obesity Myth*; Oliver, *Fat Politics*.

7   Lyons, "Prescription for Harm."

8   Raisborough, *Fat Bodies, Health and the Media*, 51–70.

9   Thanks to my hubby for being the first one to ask it!

10 Lindo Bacon and Amee Severson, "Fat Is Not the Problem—Fat Stigma Is," *Scientific American*, July 8, 2019, https://blogs.scientificamerican.com/observations/fat-is-not-the-problem-fat-stigma-is/.

11 "Ellen Maud Bennett," *Times Colonist*, May 11, 2018, https://www.legacy.com/obituaries/timescolonist/obituary.aspx?n=ellen-maud-bennett&pid=189588876.

12 I say "even more" because poverty itself is absolutely a killer. While there are many public health studies that name poverty as one of the most salient social determinants of health, here is a study that pairs this with issues of ob*sity: Medvedyuk, Ali, and Raphael, "Ideology, Obesity, and the Social Determinants of Health."

13 Stern, "Forced Sterilization."

14 Kathleen LeBesco, "Quest for a Cause: The Fat Gene, The Gay Gene, and the New Eugenics," in Rothblum and Solovay, *The Fat Studies Reader*, 65–74.

15 See ibid. LeBesco likens this to the worrisome quest to isolate "the gay gene" and the potential eugenic choices that might result.

16 Ibid., 59.

17 Raisborough, *Fat Bodies, Health and the Media*, 51–76.

18 Susan Sontag, "Disease as Political Metaphor," *The New York Review of Books*, February 23, 1978, https://www.nybooks.com/articles/1978/02/23/disease-as-political-metaphor/.

19 Cooper, *Fat Activism*, 185.

20 Wolf, *The Beauty Myth*, 94.

21 Bless you for leading the way, Washington State! In 2019 ob*sity became a new protected class in Washington State. Michigan has protected workers against weight-based discrimination since 1976, though that law has limited room for enforcement. Rebecca Puhl, "Weight Discrimination is Rampant. Yet in Most Places It's Still Legal," *The Washington Post*, June 21, 2019, https://www.washingtonpost.com/outlook/weight-discrimination-is-rampant-yet-in-most-places-its-still-legal/2019/06/21/f958613e-9394-11e9-b72d-d56510fa753e_story.html.

22 Bacon, *Health at Every Size*.

23 Erdman Farrell, *Fat Shame*, 11–13.

24 Ibid.

25 Bacon, *Health at Every Size*. Please note that Lindo has a complicated relationship with the Health at Every Size movement. Many HAES concepts first originated within the Fat Underground, a fat feminist movement in 1970s Los Angeles that identified and fought medical anti-fat bias. The Fat Underground seeded the wider Fat Liberation activist movement and HAES undercurrents were maintained therein, often by fat women of color. Lindo published their *Health at Every Size* book using the HAES moniker as their title and their book became quite popular. Lindo also took speaking engagements and led trainings using their HAES approach, garnering further popularity and becoming arguably the most well-known HAES advocate (see their website lindobacon.com). Lindo is a thin, white person, and their appropriation of HAES as the title of their book has led many to assume that Lindo is the

founder of the HAES movement, which they are not. This is especially problematic because the HAES framework as proposed by Lindo in their book implicitly supports weight-loss culture with measures that revert to reducing one's size. The Association for Size Diversity and Health (ASDAH) was founded in 2003 as an international community of fat activists and health care providers and has trademarked "Health at Every Size" in order to keep the principles of the movement in community hands, rather than with any one individual. Though publicly acknowledging some of the issues with their appropriation of HAES, Lindo has been unwilling to step back as a speaker or leader and is currently planning a new "fifteenth anniversary" edition of their HAES book, which will further bolster their visibility at a time when fat activists of color are being centered in the Fat Liberation movement. Fat activists of color have called out HAES trainings and workshops as spaces dominated by thin, white women decrying diet culture while still maintaining their thin/white privilege and sidelining larger and non-white HAES practitioners. This "thin/white-washing" of HAES has been caused, in part, by Lindo's appropriative actions. ASDAH recently revoked Lindo's membership and published communications indicating some examples of Lindo's problematic behavior. See ASDAH, "Holding Lindo Bacon Accountable for Repeated Harm in the Fat Liberation & HAES Communities," ASDAH website, March 10, 2022, https://asdah. org/lindo-accountability/. See also Marquisele Mercedes, "I Will Never Work with You," *Patreon*, March 8, 2022, https://www.patreon.com/posts/63524845.

26 The Fat Underground was a movement in 1970s Los Angeles to change the stigma of fatness within medical culture. The group used provocative rhetoric such as, "Doctors are the enemy. Weight loss is genocide." See Sara Golda Bracha Fishman, "Life in the Fat Underground," *Radiance Magazine* (Winter 1998), http://www.radiancemagazine.com/issues/1998/winter_98/fat_underground.html.

27 ASDAH, "What We Do," https://asdah.org/what-we-do/.

28 Louise Mansfield and Emma Rich, "Public Health Pedagogy, Border Crossing, and Physical Activity at Every Size," *Critical Public Health* 23, no. 3 (2013): 356–70, https://doi.org/10.1080/09581596.2013.783685; Jennifer Brady, Jacqui Gingras, and Lucy Aphramor, "Theorizing Health at Every Size as a Relational-Cultural Endeavor," *Critical Public Health* 23, no. 3 (2013): 345–55, http://dx.doi.org/10.1080/09581596.2013.797565.

29 Crowe, "Obesity Research."

30 David A. Frederick, A. Janet Tomiyama, Jyelyn G. Bold, and Abigail C. Saguy, "Can She Be Healthy at Her Weight? Effects of News Media Frames

on Antifat Attitudes, Dieting Intentions, and Perceived Health Risks of Obesity," *Stigma and Health* 5, no. 3 (August 2020): 247–57; Danna Ethan, Corey H. Basch, Grace Clarke Hillyer, Alyssa Berdnik, and Mary Huynh, "An Analysis of Weight Loss Articles and Advertisements in Mainstream Women's Health and Fitness Magazines," *Health Promotion Perspectives* 6, no. 2 (June 11, 2016): 80–84, https://doi.org/10.15171/hpp.2016.14.

31 Erdman Farrell, *Fat Shame*, 12.

32 Aubrey Gordon, writing as Your Fat Friend, "We Have to Stop Thinking of Being 'Healthy' As Being Morally Better," *Self*, August 7, 2020, https://www.self.com/story/healthism.

33 Gordon, *What We Don't Talk About When We Talk About Fat*, 10–11.

34 Robert Crawford, "Healthism and the Medicalization of Everyday Life," *International Journal of Health Services* 10, no. 3 (1980): 365–88, https://doi.org/10.2190/3h2h-3xjn-3kay-g9ny.

35 Caryn N. Bell, Jordan Kerr, and Jessica L. Young, "Associations Between Obesity, Obesogenic Environments, and Structural Racism Vary by County-Level Racial Composition," *International Journal of Environmental Research and Public Health* 16 (2019), https://doi.org/10.3390/ijerph16050861; Paula M. Brochu, "Weight Stigma is a Modifiable Risk Factor," *Journal of Adolescent Health* 63, no. 3 (September 2018): 267–68, https://doi.org/10.1016/j.jadohealth.2018.06.016.

36 Crawford, "Healthism."

37 Healthist bias is also at work when my doctors regularly instruct me to "eat less" without considering whether I eat enough in the first place. Fat people can and do have eating disorders—usually learned behaviors from diets and weight-loss culture—but these disorders often go untreated because of patients' larger sizes. See Tatjana Almuli, "The Pain of Having an Eating Disorder When You're Fat," *Vice*, October 9, 2020, https://www.vice.com/en/article/939d7p/eating-disorder-when-fat-binge-eating-atypical-anorexia.

38 An entire peer-reviewed journal has arisen on the topic of how stigmas of all sorts affect peoples' health and wellness, entitled *Stigma and Health*. Patrick W. Corrigan, ed., *Stigma and Health* (American Psychological Association, 2015–present), https://psycnet.apa.org/PsycARTICLES/journal/sah/6/2.

39 Tovar, *You Have the Right to Remain Fat*, 75–88.

40 Resmaa Menakem, *My Grandmother's Hands: Racialized Trauma and the Pathway to Mending Our Hearts and Bodies* (Las Vegas, NV: Central Recovery Press, 2017); Bengt B. Arnetz and Rolf Ekman, eds., *Stress in Health and Disease* (Weinheim: Wiley-VCH, 2006).

41 Peter Muennig, "The Body Politic: The Relationship Between Stigma and Obesity-Associated Disease," *BMC Public Health* 8, no. 128 (2008), https://doi.org/10.1186/1471-2458-8-128.

42 Vincent L. Wester, Steven W. J. Lamberts, Elisabeth F. C. van Rossum, "Advances in the Assessment of Cortisol Exposure and Sensitivity," *Current Opinion in Endocrinology, Diabetes, and Obesity* 21, no. 4 (2014): 306–11.

43 Ya-Ke Wu and Diane C. Berry, "Impact of Weight Stigma on Physiological and Psychological Health Outcomes for Overweight and Obese Adults: A Systematic Review," *Journal of Advanced Nursing* 74, no. 5 (2018): 1030–42.

44 Medvedyuk, Ali, and Raphael, "Ideology, Obesity, and the Social Determinants of Health."

Chapter 11: Disbelief Is a Starting Place

1   Mundy, *Dispensing with the Truth*, 33–51.

2   J. Eric Oliver, *Fat Politics: The Real Story Behind America's Obesity Epidemic* (New York: Oxford University Press, 2006), 1–5; Katherine M. Flegal, et al., "Association of All-Cause Mortality."

3   Brown, *Body of Truth*, 102–108.

4   Katherine M. Flegal, "The Obesity Wars and the Education of a Researcher: A Personal Account," *Progress in Cardiovascular Diseases*, June 15, 2021, https://doi.org/10.1016/j.pcad.2021.06.009.

5   Amy, Aalborg, Lyons, et al., "Barriers to Routine Gynecological Cancer Screening for White and African-American Obese Women."

6   Hobbes, "Everything You Know about Obesity Is Wrong."

7   It's a sad truth that thinner people are listened to more readily in conversations about weight bias than fat people are. No matter how solid their research is, straight-sized experts have never experienced the lived reality of fatness, which is a limitation to their understanding of the subject matter.

8   These are in no particular order other than my stream of thought. And this list is nowhere near exhaustive of the wonderful fat writers taking

on the activism and cultural criticism necessary to dismantle anti-fatness in society.

Chapter 12: Original Sin, Self-Control, and "Good" Christian Bodies

1   "Original Sin" is a theological concept stemming from the Genesis story of the "Fall," where Eve disobeys God and eats from the Tree of Knowledge, which God has expressly forbidden. This first "sin" originates a host of punishments from God including humanity's expulsion from Paradise. St. Augustine was the first to name the lasting consequences "Original Sin," claiming that everyone is born inherently sinful through the corrupted bodily lineage of Eve. See Ernesto Bonaiuti and Giorgio La Piana, "The Genesis of St. Augustine's Idea of Original Sin," *The Harvard Theological Review* 10, no. 2 (April 1917): 159–75.

2   The "eschaton" (there's a good Scrabble word for you) is another word for what Paul considered the culminating event in history—Jesus's foretold return that would usher in God's great judgment of souls and a new heavenly realm. Paul's philosophies have shaped Christian faith for millennia, but while reading his epistles, it's important to remember that most were written while expecting Christ's imminent return within his own lifetime.

3   Susan Bardo's wonderful essay "*Anorexia Nervosa: P*sychopathology as the Crystallization of Culture" suggests that the "metaphysics" of anorexia (such as the desire to be freed from bodily hungers altogether) reflect dualistic notions of freeing soul from body. Bardo names Plato, Augustine, and Descartes as a three-part chain of highly influential Western dualistic philosophers whose demand for mental/spiritual control over bodily appetites seeded Christianity's anti-body ethic.

4   Theologians who wrote within the first few centuries after Jesus's earthly ministry whose writings deeply influenced the growing Christian faith.

5   "Complementarianism" is a theological view that arises in each of the three Abrahamic religions, Judaism, Islam, and Christianity. It asserts that women and men were created by God to perform different but complementary roles in the household, religious life, and society. While men are assumed to be protectors and leaders, women should be nurturers and a helper to their man in whatever ways he chooses. Religious sects that uphold this theology often do not allow women certain leadership roles at the head of their communities and put great emphasis on female bodily purity, marriage, and fertility as women's most God-designed functions. Of course, the power dynamic at work in complementarian understandings of gender is troubling. It has led to

patriarchal culture full of misogyny, abuse, and second-class citizenship in both society and religious life for women. This ideal also reinforces a binary understanding of gender and heterosexual relationships that leaves no room for alternative expressions of gender, sexuality, or identity.

6   Lisa Isherwood and Elizabeth Stewart, *Introducing Body Theology* (Sheffield, England: Sheffield Academic Press, 1998), 15.

7   Michelle Mary Lelwica, *Shameful Bodies: Religion and the Culture of Physical Improvement* (London: Bloomsbury, 2017), 25–27.

8   Tertullian, *De Cultu Feminarum* (Book I, Chapter I), trans S. Thelwall (1869).

9   St. Jerome, *Against Jovinianus* (N.p.: Amazon Digital Services LLC—KDP Print US, 2019).

10 Isherwood and Stewart, *Introducing Body Theology*, 18.

11 Saint Augustine, "Letter to Laetus," in *The Works of Saint Augustine: Letters 211–270*, ed. Augustinian Heritage Institute, trans. Roland Teske (New York: New York City Press, 2005), 169.

12 John Chrysostom, "Homily 9 on 1 Timothy," trans. Philip Schaff, in *Nicene and Post-Nicene Fathers, First Series,* vol. 13 (Buffalo, NY: Christian Literature Publishing, 1889).

13 Lelwica, *Shameful Bodies*, 26.

14 Ibid.

15 Wolf, *The Beauty Myth*, 93.

16 Augustine, *On the Trinity, Book 12, Chapter 7, Paragraph 10.*

17 Rudolph M. Bell, *Holy Anorexia* (Chicago: University of Chicago Press, 1985), 54–83.

18 Richard Klein, "Fat Beauty," in Braziel and LeBesco, *Bodies Out of Bounds*, 33. However, other scholars of church history suggest that fasting was no more prevalent in religious women than religious men of the day, and that it was not universally appreciated as a spiritual practice. Some church leaders accused long-fasting women of witchcraft or possession. See Walter Vandereycken and Ron van Deth, *From Fasting Saints to Anorexic Girls: The History of Self-Starvation* (New York: New York University Press, 1994).

19 By the fourth century, "gluttony" was already characterized as one of the "principle vices" of humankind. St. John Cassian, a monastic theologian of the day wrote, "There are eight principal vices that attack humankind. The first is gluttony, which means the voraciousness of the belly." He proceeded to give principles of eating so that one did not endanger their spirituality: "Food is to be taken insofar as it supports our life, but not to the extent of enslaving us to the impulses of desire. To eat moderately and reasonably is to keep the body in health, not to deprive it of holiness . . . No one whose stomach is full can fight mentally against the demon of unchastity." Note here a conflation of health and holiness on the one hand and gluttony and sexuality on the other. Cassian's "principle vices" became popular themes as other theologians riffed on these "troublesome" aspects of the human condition. Thomas Aquinas, in particular, spent a great deal of time on the nuances of gluttony in his tome *Summa Theologica*. See St. John Cassian, *The Monastic Institutes: On the Training of a Monk and the Eight Deadly Sins*, trans. Jerome Bertram (London: Saint Austin Press, 1999); Thomas Aquinas, *Summa Theologica* (Christian Classics, 1948). For a secondary source discussion, see also Griffith, *Born Again Bodies*, 62, 219–20; Hillel Schwartz, *Never Satisfied*, 92–95, 159–62.

20 Lelwica, *Shameful Bodies*, 27–29, 67–72.

21 Ibid., 27, 67–69.

22 Ibid., 27–28.

23 In chapter 14 I will discuss an alternative narrative where Jesus's healing was not for the sake of individual assimilation but societal liberation.

24 Lelwica, *Shameful Bodies*, 67–72.

25 See Matthew 9:22, Mark 10:52, and Luke 17:19.

26 See John 8:11 and John 5:14.

27 Nancy L. Eiesland, *The Disabled God: Toward a Liberatory Theology of Disability* (Nashville, TN: Abingdon Press, 1994), 71; Lelwica, *Shameful Bodies*, 67–72.

28 Eiesland, *The Disabled God*, 74.

29 Sadly, this is not just a historical issue but a current one. Those with mental and physical disabilities still find barriers to their ordination in some denominations. Even more frequently, disabled people have

limited access within church buildings themselves. Churches often do not have the ramps or elevators necessary, for example, to inhabit the pulpit while in a wheelchair. Lelwica, *Shameful Bodies*, 68.

30 Ibid., 77.

31 Eiesland, *The Disabled God*, 72.

32 Council on Developmental Disabilities, "Parallels in Time: A History of Developmental Disabilities" (Minnesota Governor's Council on Developmental Disabilities, 2021), https://mn.gov/mnddc/parallels/index.html.

33 The word "crip," as shorthand for the word "crippled," is being reclaimed in disability communities the same way that "queer" has been in gay communities, and the overlap between the two communities includes the challenge to culturally understood "normalcy." See McRuer, *Crip Theory* and Hanebutt and Mueller, "Disability Studies, Crip Theory, and Education."

34 Eiesland, *The Disabled God*; Sharon V. Betcher, *Spirit and the Politics of Disablement* (Minneapolis, MN: Fortress Press, 2007).

35 There is a complex relationship between disability politics and fat politics. Fat activists have sometimes avoided the moniker of "disability" as they fight for fatness to be seen as a "normal" body type rather than an exceptional one. In the same way, some disabled activists see fatness not as an ingrained identity but as a mutable characteristic, one that is not formed genetically but by one's inability to control their gluttony. Unfortunately, both of these arguments miss the real opportunity to align efforts toward body liberation in a wider sense, an ultimate goal that would serve both groups. For more nuance in these arguments see LeBesco, *Revolting Bodies*, 74–84; Cooper, *Fat Activism*, 162–70, 184–88; Solovay, *Tipping the Scales of Justice*, 128–70.

36 Irina Metzler, "Disabled Children: Birth Defects, Causality and Guilt," in *Medicine, Religion and Gender in Medieval Culture*, ed. Naoë Kukita Yoshikawa (Cambridge: D.S. Brewer, 2015), 161–80.

37 Louise Gosbell, "'As Long as It's Healthy': What Can We Learn from Early Christianity's Resistance to Infanticide and Exposure," *ABC Religion and Ethics*, December 18, 2020, https://www.abc.net.au/religion/early-christianitys-resistance-to-infanticide-and-exposure/10898016.

38 Or any other gender expression beyond the binary.

39 Gosbell, "As Long as It's Healthy."

40 Ibid.

The Parable of the Weeds

1   I have searched and searched for this poem and cannot find it again.
I wonder if perhaps I dreamt it or if it's not yet written at all. Surely, if
someone knows this poem and can find it, you'll please be in touch with
me so I can finally put my mind at ease.

Chapter 13: Jesus and the Reluctant Saints of Fat Liberation

1   Cooper, *Fat Activism*, 33–34.

2   For an analysis of how fatness is portrayed and understood according
to media representations, see Raisborough, *Fat Bodies, Health and the
Media.*

3   Erdman Farrell, *Fat Shame*, 137–71.

4   Ryan Fraser, "Your Body is a Temple," *The Jackson Sun*, June 19,
2015, https://www.jacksonsun.com/story/life/faith/2015/06/19/
body-temple/29162173/.

5   This has been my M.O. since late high school. If I sense someone's
fatphobic judgment, I rebel by eating more as a performance of my
disregard for their concern. On the one hand, this makes me feel better
because I know how much it irks them. But what I've come to realize is
that this still roots my food decisions in their hands, albeit the reverse
of what they'd want me to choose. Psychologically this is an anger
response, a rebellious reaction to the restrictive dieting of my youth.
I'm currently trying to emerge from this pattern into one that gives
me more personal agency around my food choices. Ignoring other
people's fatphobic concerns entirely, I'm starting to ask myself, "okay,
do I want this brownie or not?" If I do, awesome. I eat it for me, not in
defiance of others. If I don't want it, fine also. It was my choice not to
eat it, not a rebellion against their healthist concerns. I'm navigating
this struggle daily and it's central to my healing. "Healing" for me
would not be defined by weight loss but by making my body *mine* again,
instead of an object of either diet culture's concerns or praise. This
would be an individual signpost on the long road of collective, societal
dismantling of anti-fat bias. I know this is a deep dive into my personal
psychology, which may seem strange. However, I'm choosing to name
this experience in case someone else suffers similarly and needs to feel
camaraderie in their struggle.

6   Aubrey Gordon, writing as Your Fat Friend, "I Will Not Help You Hate
Your Body," *Medium*, August 12, 2019, https://humanparts.medium.com/

your-bad-body-image-doesnt-end-with-you-6014f03746d0.

7   Aubrey Gordon, writing as Your Fat Friend, "It's Time to Retire 'You're Not Fat, You're Beautiful!'," *Self*, January 19, 2021, https://www.self.com/story/not-fat-beautiful.

Chapter 14: Jesus Heals a Woman

1   This "identity-first language" may feel awkward to some readers, but it is promoted by progressive disability activism. Cara Liebowitz, "I Am Disabled: On Identity-First versus People-First Language," *The Body is Not an Apology*, March 20, 2015, https://thebodyisnotanapology.com/magazine/i-am-disabled-on-identity-first-versus-people-first-language/.

2   We need to get away from seeing bodies as "normal" or "not normal" and instead see them as individually dignified and agentic people with unique needs. So, when I use "norm" here and elsewhere, I mean "societal norm" and am not advocating for one particular "norm," because there is no such thing.

3   Shelly Rambo, *Resurrecting Wounds: Living in the Afterlife of Trauma* (Waco, TX: Baylor University Press, 2017), 71–107.

4   Rambo, *Resurrecting Wounds*, 73.

5   Ibid., 71–107.

6   Ibid., 73, 93–94, 106–107.

7   Ibid., 106–107.

8   For a history of how racism and anti-fatness were perpetuated alongside one another in the colonization of America, see Strings, *Fearing the Black Body*.

9   Rambo, *Resurrecting Wounds*, 63–69, 124–25.

10   Ibid., 102, 106–107.

11   The full account of this narrative can be found in the gospel of John: John 20:24–29.

12   Mark 5:34.

13   This connotes what Charlotte Cooper calls the "headless fatty" image, which is very prevalent in the media. Charlotte Cooper, "Headless Fatties."

14 Rambo, *Resurrecting Wounds*, 73.

15 Strings, *Fearing the Black Body*.

The Pantry

1   Many studies link restrictive dieting in one's youth to poorer overall health behaviors in adulthood, as well as psychological issues including depression, anxiety, perfectionism, and eating disorders. Researchers are coming to understand what fat activists have said all along: the weight stigma enacted on people is what makes them unwell, not their adipose tissue. And children, who have not yet formed their sense of self, internalize negative weight messages maybe even more than their adult counterparts. See Virginia Sole-Smith, "The Last Thing Fat Kids Need," *Slate*, April 19, 2021, https://slate.com/technology/2021/04/child-separation-weight-stigma-diets.html; A. Janet Tomiyama, Deborah Carr, Ellen M. Granberg, Brenda Major, Eric Robinson, Angelina R. Sutin, and Alexandra Brewis, "How and Why Weight Stigma Drives the Obesity 'Epidemic' and Harms Health," *BMC Medicine* 16, no. 123 (2018), https://doi.org/10.1186/s12916-018-1116-5; Rebecca M. Puhl and Janet D. Latner, "Stigma, Obesity, and the Health of the Nation's Children," *Psychological Bulletin of the American Psychological Association* 133, no. 4 (July 2007): 557–80, https://psycnet.apa.org/buy/2007-09203-001.

2   Rebecca Puhl and Young Suh, "Health Consequences of Weight Stigma: Implications for Obesity Prevention and Treatment," *Current Obesity Reports* 4 (April 2015): 182–90, https://doi.org/10.1007/s13679-015-0153-z.

Chapter 15: God Becomes Flesh

1   Theologians Rita Nakashima Brock and Rebecca Parker suggest that this is the "apex of the Christian proclamation: that Christ has reopened paradise by his incarnation and resurrection, not by the Crucifixion." How might a reclaiming of incarnation, rather than crucifixion, change our theology and lived spirituality? See Rita Nakashima Brock and Rebecca Ann Parker, *Saving Paradise: How Christianity Traded Love of This World for Crucifixion and Empire* (Boston: Beacon Press, 2008), 466.

Chapter 16: Embracing the Gospel of Fat Liberation Even When We Don't Feel It

1   Cooper, *Fat Activism*, 17.

2   Denny, "What It's Like to Be Transgender and Face Dysphoria and Body Dysmorphia at the Same Time," *Allure Magazine*, February 27, 2019, https://www.allure.com/story/transgender-body-dysmorphia-gender-dysphoria-effects.

3   Fancis Ray White, "Fat and Trans: Towards a New Theorization of Gender in Fat Studies," in Pausé and Taylor, *The Routledge Internaonal Handbook of Fat Studies*, 78–87.

4   Cooper, *Fat Activism*, 17.

5   Nina Mackert and Jürgen Martschukat, "Introduction: Fat Agency," *Body Politics* 3 (2015): 5–11, http://bodypolitics.de/de/wp-content/uploads/2016/01/Heft_5_01_Mackert_Martschukat_Intro_End-1.pdf.

6   Ryan Benson, the first *Biggest Loser* winner in 2004, described fasting and dehydrating his body to the point of urinating blood (a sign of kidney disease) prior to the finale show. Edward Wyatt, "On 'The Biggest Loser,' Health Can Take Back Seat," *The New York Times*, November 24, 2009, https://www.nytimes.com/2009/11/25/business/media/25loser.html. See also Sophie Gilbert, "The Retrograde Shame of *The Biggest Loser*," *The Atlantic*, January 29, 2020, https://www.theatlantic.com/culture/archive/2020/01/the-retrograde-shame-of-the-biggest-loser/605713/.

7   "Good Fatty and Bad Fatty Explained," *Fat Positive Cooperative*, December 12, 2018, https://fatpositivecooperative.com/2018/12/12/good-fatty-and-bad-fatty-explained/. For a discussion of the healthism inherent in being a "good fatty" see Gibson, "Health(ism) at Every Size."

8   Aubrey Gordon's essay on flying while fat is a must read. Aubrey Gordon, writing as Your Fat Friend, "A Letter from the Fat Person on Your Flight," *Medium: Human Parts*, October 9, 2017, https://humanparts.medium.com/a-letter-from-the-fat-person-on-your-flight-b0ceb1407c61.

9   The average airline seat has shrunk from a pitch of thirty-five inches and width of 18.5 inches forty years ago to its current average pitch of thirty-one inches and width of seventeen inches. Stephanie Sarkis, "Airlines' Seat Pitch Gets Shorter and Passengers Reach Their Limit," *Forbes*, February 24, 2020, https://www.forbes.com/sites/stephaniesarkis/2020/02/24/airlines-seat-pitch-gets-shorter-and-passengers-reach-their-limits/?sh=2ee3ead4441a.

10 Celeste Hamilton Dennis, "How a Stock Photography Project is Confronting Anti-Fat Bias," *Yes Magazine*, December 17, 2019, https://www.yesmagazine.org/social-justice/2019/12/17/stock-photos-fat-bias.

Chapter 17: Never Leaving Paradise

1   A younger version of Girl Scouts.

2   The idea that women were only created to "complete" men and to serve

under male leadership. See the discussion of complementarianism in chapter 12.

3   There are plenty of biblical passages that undermine women, their agency, and their bodies, not just the second Creation narrative in Genesis. And so, some might rightfully suggest that my focus on this one passage is limited, which I fully admit. However, this second Creation narrative is the passage that pegs the origin of humanity's sin and problems on Eve, on women's disobedience, forever lending an argument to any church leader who places controls on women's bodies. This makes it a critical passage, and its interpretation through the centuries should be interrogated accordingly.

4   Rita Nakashima Brock and Rebecca Parker, "This Present Paradise," *UU World*, July 14, 2008, https://www.uuworld.org/articles/ early-christians-emphasized-paradise-not-crucifixion.

5   Nakashima Brock and Parker, *Saving Paradise*, 29–30.

6   Ibid., 30–31.

7   Ibid., 90–91.

8   Ibid., xix.

9   This is the description of the painting employed in *The New Yorker*'s announcement of an interactive website in which viewers can take an in-depth electronic look at the painting's entire tryptic, which physically resides at the Prado in Madrid, Spain. Here is the interactive website, which was erected in 2016 by Bosch's hometown upon the 500th anniversary of his death in 1516: *Jheronimus Bosch—The Garden of Earthly Delights,* https://archief.ntr.nl/tuinderlusten/en.html#. And here is the article about its release: Alexandra Schwartz, "Click Here to Visit Hell: An Interactive 'Garden of Earthly Delights,'" *The New Yorker*, April 12, 2016, https://www.newyorker.com/culture/rabbit-holes/ click-here-to-visit-hell-an-interactive-garden-of-earthly-delights.

10 A triptych is a three-paneled painting or relief that is hinged so it can hold together. Opened up, it can be used to decorate a church's altar table.

11 Hans Belting, *Hieronymus Bosch Garden of Earthly Delights* (Munich: Prestel, 2018), 71–73.

12 Ibid., 74.

13 Ibid., 89.

ACKNOWLEDGEMENTS

I have one big, fat community surrounding me, and for that I am exceedingly grateful.

First, to Rachel Hackenberg and Katie Martin at The Pilgrim Press, whose faith in this project was immediate, unwavering, and unexpected. The shock of your counsel has bolstered me in ways I'm still realizing. Thanks for believing in *Fat Church* from the very beginning. Thanks also to the infinitely patient Diane Hackenberg, editor extraordinaire, who improved greatly the structure and readability of this work, sharing of her personal self along the way. Adam Bresnahan offered the final fine-toothed comb across the book's grammatical surface. I feel very lucky to have worked with this team at The Pilgrim Press.

My husband, Chad Kidd, deserves ample praise for being my biggest supporter. Hon, you read every draft, you were my sounding board for every errant idea, and you fed both my body and ego when self-doubts arose. Your trust in my ability to do this work is part of what got me here. "Thank you, and I love you" seem not nearly enough to express my gratitude for all that you are to me. My Uncle Bob Bailey has become a fat activist in his own right! He even surprised me with the gorgeous painting that is the basis of this book's cover art. I have trusted his counsel my whole life long and am grateful that our friendship has deepened to a point where I can't tell uncle from brother from friend. Uncle Bob, thank you for being my favorite. Alongside them, my extended family has seen me through by their love: Breon Dunigan and Liam Bailey; Lyndsie, Josh, Noah, and Jeremiah Blakely; Sharla and Chip Hall; and Chuck Kidd.

I am indebted to those who offered their time and energy to read early drafts of this manuscript and provide invaluable feedback. Alexandra Adams, Linda Jerrett, Robyn Kinch, Vince Tango, Lisa Gibbs, and Sangwon Yang, thank you for being gentle and compassionate guides in my life, for your wisdom, and for all the irreverent comments in the margins. The incomparable Bill Gillis—fellow writer, Southern lore enthusiast, and my favorite storyteller for two decades—thank you for the straight talk. And also, the gay talk. You are my respite from ridiculousness and I'm so grateful for you. Early and ongoing conversations with Megan Hornbeek-Allen unearthed in us both the gumption to want more. Love you, Dorothy.

I am lucky to have many friends who are like family to me. They have offered jokes, cocktails, prayers, and/or advice in the more challenging moments of this project. Heather Huskey and Lea Yerby are sages and companions, essential to me through every important milestone since college, including this one. I am in awe of how far our Awesome, Party of Three, has come. Thank you to Shelly Rambo, whose humanity, wit, and theology inspire me in equal measure; to Michael Yuille, who reminds me of the power of trusting one's own rudder; and to the whole Buckman-Rambo clan—Jody, Ty, Helena, and Wyeth—treasures all. Andy Linscott is my chosen brother, confessor, and confidant. Thank you for always picking up when I call. Thank you to Mike and Diana Duke and Debi Eley for rootedness and joy in homegoing, to Yara González-Justiniano for truth-telling wisdom and for always cultivating beauty, to Pippa Mpunzwana for memory-keeping and being a model of hopefulness, to Kristen McCarthy for constant delight and all the memes, to Pallu Reddy for never outgrowing me or our beloved mixed tapes, and to Annie Britton and Terry Schwennesen for steadfast compassion and companionship. Thank you to those friends who are also dear colleagues, who made room for me to take the breaks necessary to finish this work, especially Gretchen Brown, M Damm, and Bryan Stone. And thanks to the inimitable Jason Juan Rodriguez for (real talk) always keeping me afloat. I'm grateful for the weekly plunge outside of reality that my Progress adventuring crew provides, and for all the belly laughs. Josh Blakely,

Josh Hasler and Laura Carlson Hasler, Blake Fox and Kaitlyn Martin Fox, and Chad and Kendra Moore are some of the best people I know. I'm in awe of their wisdom (checks). I'm also glad to call some of my dear friends my spiritual guides. Holly Benzenhafer, Wendy Miller Olapade, Emelia Attridge, and Kathryn House, you are four horsewomen of the patriarchy's apocalypse.

Finally, to my parents, Bill and Mona Bailey, who I knew as Mama and Papa. And to Gregory Bailey, who I knew as Daddy. Thank you for loving me so well, and for being proud of the ways I both upkept and diverged from our family values. You loved all of me, and I love all of you. Forever.